ROUTLEDGE LIBRARY EDITIONS:
NURSE EDUCATION AND
NURSING CARE

Volume 5

RESEARCH INTO NURSE EDUCATION

RESEARCH INTO
NURSE EDUCATION

Edited by
BRYN D. DAVIS

Routledge
Taylor & Francis Group

LONDON AND NEW YORK

First published in 1983 by Croom Helm Ltd.

This edition first published in 2026
by Routledge
4 Park Square, Milton Park, Abingdon, Oxon OX14 4RN

and by Routledge
605 Third Avenue, New York, NY 10158

Routledge is an imprint of the Taylor & Francis Group, an informa business

British Library Cataloguing in Publication Data
A catalogue record for this book is available from the British Library

ISBN: 978-1-041-11658-5 (Set)
ISBN: 978-1-041-11154-2 (Volume 5) (hbk)
ISBN: 978-1-041-11156-6 (Volume 5) (pbk)
ISBN: 978-1-003-65853-5 (Volume 5) (ebk)

DOI: 10.4324/9781003658535

Publisher's Note
The publisher has gone to great lengths to ensure the quality of this reprint but points out that some imperfections in the original copies may be apparent.

Disclaimer
The publisher has made every effort to trace copyright holders and would welcome correspondence from those they have been unable to trace.

Research into Nurse Education

Edited by Bryn D. Davis

CROOM HELM
London & Canberra

© 1983 Bryn D. Davis
Croom Helm Ltd; Provident House, Burrell Row,
Beckenham, Kent BR3 1AT

British Library Cataloguing in Publication Data

Research into nurse education
   1 Nursing—Study and teaching
   I Davis, Bryn D.
   610 73'07'11   RT71
    ISBN 0-7099-0825-3

Printed and bound in Great Britain
by Billing & Sons Limited, Worcester.

CONTENTS

LIST OF CONTRIBUTORS

John A. Birch, PhD, MEd, SRN, RNT,
Chief Nursing Officer, North Lincolnshire Health District, Lincoln.

Senga Bond, PhD, MSc, BA, RGN,
Nursing Research Liaison Officer, Northern Regional Health Authority.

Ena Chakrabarty, BA, Dip Lib, ALA,
Librarian, Wolfson School of Nursing of Westminster, London.

Bryn D. Davis, BSc, SRN, RMN, RNT,
Deputy Director, Nursing Research Unit, Department of Nursing Studies, University of Edinburgh.

Marjorie Gott, PhD, BA, SRN, HV, Cert Ed, RNT,
Lecturer in Nursing Studies, Department of Social Studies, Trent Polytechnic, Nottingham.

Barbara R. Lewis, PhD,
Senior Lecturer, Department of Management Sciences, University of Manchester Institute of Science and Technology.

Margaret E. Ogier, PhD, BSc, SRN, SCM, DipN, RNT,
Senior Tutor, Emma Ferbrache School of Nursing, Princess Elizabeth Hospital, Guernsey.

Helen D. Orton, BA(Hons), MPhil,
Principal Lecturer, Department of Health Studies, Sheffield City Polytechnic.

John Sheahan, MSc, MEd, DipFE, SRN, RMN, RNT, FRSH,
Principal Lecturer in Nursing, Faculty of Education, Huddersfield Polytechnic.

John C.A. Wells, BA, MA, SRN, RMN, RNT,
Deputy Director of Education of the Royal College of Nursing and Vice Principal of the Institute of Advanced Nursing Education, Royal College of Nursing of the United Kingdom, London.

GENERAL INTRODUCTION

This book consists of a collection of chapters, written by different authors, reporting the main findings and implications of research or development in nurse education. Each chapter has individual merit, exploring various questions which challenge nurse educationalists. The individual chapters can be read in isolation, for each makes a separate contribution to the sum of knowledge regarding this subject.

As a collection, it is felt that links between the chapters and themes and findings from them add up to a more complex and revealing perspective. These links lead to a view of nurse education which confirms the need to deal with learners as individuals with their own levels of ability, traits, vulnerabilities, ways of looking at nurse training and of coping with it. This requires tutors who are prepared and supported so that they can deliver an educational process which includes an active role for individual learners, with experiences and supervision in the clinical setting to provide the optimum environment for the process of becoming a nurse.

It is hoped, therefore, that the book will be read at two levels. As a series of individual research reports, the reader can select those of particular relevance or interest. As a volume on research into nurse education, presenting evidence from the various chapters, it is hoped that the book will also be read in order to study the links between them. To this end, this general introduction, the section introductions, and the conclusion offer a supporting structure to the individual chapters. Building from these bricks a whole can be built which is more than the respective parts. This whole is a statement about nurse education, drawing on the evidence provided by the authors of the chapters and evidence from other recent work and developments to provide an argument concerning the future direction of the education and training of nurses.

The book has been written for people who are involved in nurse education, which includes people working as lecturers, tutors, clinical teachers, on nursing courses in schools of nursing, colleges and universities. Also included are those who, while working as practitioners in clinical areas in hospital and community, provide examples by words and deeds. It is also hoped that those who are in positions of decision and policy making concerning the systems and organisation of nurse

1

education will find much of interest and value. Finally, however, it is hoped that this book will be read by nurse learners themselves, for there is a great need for nurses to be more aware of the dynamics of the system they have entered, so that their role in the process may be more informed.

In order to set the various chapters in context, there now follows a brief historical review of the development of nurse training and of the associated research. From this it will be seen that the present trends in nurse education research arise historically in concerns that have troubled the nurse education system since the first surveys were undertaken, and before that in the disputes that surrounded the setting up of the General Nursing Councils (GNCs) in 1919.

The development of nurse training, over the last three-quarters of a century, has been mainly in response to two main pressures. These were the pressure to maintain and, if possible, improve standards of nursing, and the pressure to reduce shortages and to provide an adequate nursing service. Attitudes involving a need to provide care for the sick, and the discipline felt necessary for the provision of a skilled profession, keystones of the developing nursing service, reflect, in many ways, the social and cultural background of the Victorian middle classes, and of Florence Nightingale.

This sense of moral values and discipline has informed the management of the nursing services since then. The creation of the GNCs in 1919 did not resolve this dilemma, although it was the first step in the setting up of national standards. However, the lobbying power of the hospital matrons and the management committees and their concern for a steady supply of new recruits conflicted with the aims of the council. In order to maintain numbers, younger and younger recruits were employed.

Many inquiries in the 1930s and 1940s found that conditions of service were not satisfactory and recommendations for improvements in hours of work and pay, among other things, were made. Repeatedly, however, factors concerning the relationships between senior and junior nurses were shown to be important (*Lancet* Report, 1932; Athlone Report, 1939). Davies, in her review of the history of nursing (1980), commented that no-one argued that the poor resources and the incompatibility of service and educational requirements were important, although the Athlone Report in particular did recommend improvements in salaries and in working conditions. The government did not accept some of the Report's recommendations regarding the funding of hospitals and nurse training, but did act on many of the proposals. Nevertheless, nothing was done about the questions of discipline, relationships and support for the learner.

The Report of the Working Party (1947), concerned with the recruitment, training, wastage, and work of nurses, concluded that it was important to increase the numbers of trained nurses by recruiting more, and losing fewer. Wastage was related to discipline and attitudes as well as conditions of service. The results of the survey of learners undertaken for the Working Party showed that a high proportion of leavers were 'unsuitable for nurse training on intellectual or personality grounds'. The Report called for suitable selection procedures to be established.

Unfortunately, as with previous reports, the findings concerning interpersonal relationships, discipline and morale, were largely ignored. It was as if the interpretation of the findings of the survey was that, with the 'right' scheme of training, and the selection of the 'right' applicants, an adequate number of trained nurses would be provided. No attempts were made to study the effects on learners of poor morale, harsh discipline, and the lack of socio-emotional support, nor were attempts made to incorporate in the system the views of the learners, and what they thought of their training.

In a Minority Report, Cohen did point to the importance of discipline and attitudes as factors in nurse wastage (1948). He argued that blaming matrons, and exhorting them to change their ways was doomed unless they attempted to study the dynamics and interplay of relationships. Needless to say, it was the Majority Report of the Working Party (1947) which was heeded most.

However, some work was pursued in this direction, notably that described by Revans (1964) and Wieland and Leigh (1971). This work was concerned with relationships between, as well as within, various professional groups, although that of Towell (1975) concentrated on psychiatric nursing, and highlighted the learner's perspective.

The main impetus for research was centred on the search for selection criteria, on intellectual and personality parameters. In this way it was hoped that it would be possible to select the successful and reject unsuitable candidates or those who would be likely to fail. During the 1950s and 1960s and into the 1970s a wide range of tests and techniques were studied.

The later studies in the 1970s came to respect the importance of stress and of attitudes, but even here the concern was with the development of standardised tests for selection procedures, rather than as attempts to monitor and assess the social psychology, and the sociology of becoming and being a nurse.

In the USA work had begun in this direction, notably with medical students, and then with nurses (Merton *et al.*, 1957; Becker *et al.*, 1961; Olesen and Whittaker, 1968; Simpson *et al.*, 1979). These studies have recently been taken up and developed in the UK.

Other developments in the UK have been concerned with the clinical setting. The relationships between learner and teacher in this setting and the importance of the ward sister have been recognised, as has the importance of the link between classroom preparation and clinical experience. The problems of keeping up to date with recent research findings and developments, the acquisition and practice of management and teaching skills are also the focus of recent research and innovation.

These developments in research reflect, and in many ways were generated by, changes within the nursing profession itself. The last decade or so has seen quite a dynamic phase. These recent changes and developments will be considered further in the conclusion, when the implications of recent research, particularly those presented here, will be discussed.

The three sections in this volume echo the strands of research that have developed as described briefly above. The first section reflects the move from a concern with selection and screening to a concern with the social psychology of becoming a nurse. The second section concentrates on the question of teaching and learning on the ward, and the relative influence of the ward sister. The final section looks at the process of education and at the provision of resource material for the teachers and practitioners involved in the education and training of nurse learners.

The rationale for the various sections, and the choice of the individual chapters is given in a brief introduction to each section. The concluding statement, drawing together key points from each chapter, puts the whole collection in perspective and extends the developments described in this introduction into the future.

References

Athlone Report (1939) Ministry of Health, Board of Education: *Interdepartmental Committee on Nursing Services, Interim Report*, HMSO, London
Becker, H.S., Hughes, E.C., Greer, B. and Strauss, A.L. (1961) *Boys in White*, University of Chicago Press, Chicago
Davies, C. (1980) *Rewriting Nursing History*, Croom Helm, Beckenham, Kent
Lancet Report – *Report of the Commission on Nursing* (1932), *Lancet*, London
Merton, R.K., Reader, G.G. and Kendall, P.L. (eds.) (1957) *The Student Physician: Introductory Studies in the Sociology of Medical Education*, Harvard University Press, Cambridge, Mass.

Olesen, V.L. and Whittaker, E.W. (1968) *The Silent Dialogue*, Jossey Bass Inc., San Francisco

Report of the Working Party on the Recruitment and Training of Nurses (1947), HMSO, London

Report of the Working Party — Minority Report (1948), HMSO, London (Minority Report by John Cohen)

Revans, R.W. (1964) *Standards for Morale — Cause and Effect in Hospitals*, Nuffield Provincial Hospitals Trust, Oxford University Press

Simpson, I.H., Back, K., Ingles, T., Kerckhoff, A. and McKinney, J.C. (1979) *From Student to Nurse: A Longitudinal Study of Socialisation*, Cambridge University Press

Towell, D. (1975) *Understanding Psychiatric Nursing*, Royal College of Nursing, London

Wieland, G. and Leigh, H. (eds.), (1971) *Changing Hospitals — A Report on the Hospital Internal Communications Project*, Tavistock, London

Part One

STUDENT NURSES — CHARACTERISTICS AND PERCEPTIONS

INTRODUCTION

Bryn D. Davis

This first section is concerned with nurse learners and coping with the process of becoming a nurse. As has been pointed out in the general introduction, the major concern over the last few decades has been in determining criteria for the selection of new recruits. In Chapter 1, Lewis continues this theme and her study, which developed from a most valuable review of the literature in this field (Lewis and Cooper, 1976), reveals some of the problems inherent in this pursuit. Her aim was to describe entrants to nurse training, and to try to differentiate those who succeeded from those who withdrew and failed. In Chapter 2, Birch, who has also undertaken research in the same area (Birch, 1975) reports a study of the importance of one major factor (anxiety) on the learner's progress. His argument is that the ability to identify vulnerable nurses, using various testing devices, could facilitate the selection of more robust recruits, not so susceptible to withdrawal under pathological levels of stress.

Other recent studies have discussed problematic aspects of nursing. For example, Melia (1982) has reported student difficulties in coping with learner/worker conflict; the pressure of work; learning what the job is about; and the transient nature of the student nurse experience from interviews with general student nurses. There is little evidence from studies about psychiatric nurse training, but Cormack (1976) reported no ward teaching from his observational study and, from a participant-observational study, Towell (1975) concluded that 'conceptions of training, among hospital staff, tended to focus on what nurses were taught rather than what they learnt' (p.205). He argued that the students' experiences of nursing work, on different wards, determined the understandings about psychiatric nursing which were developed by them. Also reported were needs for more guidance, particularly in coping with discontinuities in experience and other difficulties encountered. Towell, like Melia (1982), stressed the importance of the student nurses' perspectives and role conceptions, in an attempt to understand the process of learning. Students in psychiatric nursing also tend to play a more independent role than general students, and to spend much time working with other junior nurses.

9

In Chapter 3, Davis argues that, notwithstanding the value of effect-ive selection, the way learners negotiate the stresses and problematic aspects of their training, and the way they see the various people available to act as resources for them, must be considered. Evidence of the active role played by the student nurses is presented which indi-cates that, however well selected the new recruits might be, they them-selves will determine, to a greater extent than might usually be ex-pected, how well they will cope. Particularly with younger, general student nurses, the process of becoming an adult is compounded with the process of becoming a nurse. This makes the situation much more dynamic and unpredictable.

The three chapters together can be seen as confirming the vulner-ability of some recruits. They also show that assessment of the vulner-ability could lead either to counselling against entering nursing or to learners being provided with the effective support of suitable resource people to meet individual levels of need as they occur. In particular the importance of ward-based staff in this is shown, and this is discussed further in Part 2 of this book.

References

Birch, J.A. (1975) *To Nurse or Not to Nurse: An Investigation into the Causes of Withdrawal During Nurse Training*, Royal College of Nursing, London

Cormack, D. (1976) *Psychiatric Nursing Observed*, Royal College of Nursing, London

Lewis, B.R. and Cooper, C.L. (1976) 'Personality measurement among nurses: a review', *International Journal of Nursing Studies, 13*, 209-29

Melia, K.M. (1982) Students' construction of nursing: a contribution to policy making? Proceedings of International Conference "Research — A Base for the Future?", Nursing Research Unit, University of Edinburgh, September 1981

Towell, D. (1975) *Understanding Psychiatric Nursing*, Royal College of Nursing, London

1 PERSONALITY AND INTELLECTUAL CHARACTERISTICS OF TRAINEE NURSES AND THEIR ASSESSMENT

Barbara R. Lewis

Introduction

A research investigation at the University of Manchester Institute of Science and Technology (UMIST) has considered the recruitment and selection of trainee nurses as a marketing problem, with attention directed towards showing the relevance of the concepts of 'markets', 'marketing communications' and 'consumer analysis'. The investigation also involved evaluative marketing research which was carried out by means of questionnaire-based surveys among recently recruited students and pupils and senior nursing personnel in schools of nursing in England and Wales (see Lewis, 1977, 1979).

An integral element of the research was the assessment of intellectual and personality characteristics of trainee nurses, along with a wide range of socio-economic and attitudinal variables. A further element involved the description of entrants to nurse training and, more importantly, an attempt to differentiate the learners who completed their training programmes and passed their examinations from those who withdrew from training and failed to become nurses. One of the research aims was to try to present a profile of the 'successful' trainee nurse, such that future recruitment and selection procedures could be directed at attracting such people into the profession, i.e. to increase the effectiveness of recruitment and selection and to reduce wastage from training and from the nursing profession.

Wastage From Nurse Training

Attrition from nurse training is of prime importance to nursing administrators and educators, and has been the theme of a considerable number of research surveys and reports (e.g. MacGuire, 1969). In the various papers, wastage data are presented together with discussion of reasons why nurses leave training and investigations of correlates of

11

wastage and success in nurse training.

Reasons for withdrawal are numerous but may be categorised as either involuntary (e.g. academic failure or disciplinary action leading to dismissal) or voluntary. Explanations for voluntary wastage, which accounts for the vast majority of leavers, are often difficult to obtain and categorise because the trainees concerned are either reluctant to discuss the situation, frequently are not available to talk to, or the reasons given are vague. However, the major reasons proffered relate to personal factors, dislike of nursing, criticisms of conditions of service (including pay), poor integration of training, bad staff-student relationships, and conditions in the hospital environment (see Brown, 1974; Cross and Hall, 1954; General Nursing Council, 1966; Revans, 1964; Singh and Smith, 1975; and Thompson, 1974).

Correlates of wastage and success in nurse training that pertain to the individual, which have been investigated over the years, include a wide range of socio-economic and demographic variables as discussed, for example, by Barr (1959), the GNC (1976), and Singh and Smith (1975); and also a number of intellectual factors, i.e. academic/educational attainment and intelligence. Previous educational attainment and intelligence of trainee nurses and their relationship with success in nurse training (i.e. ability to stay the course, pass the examinations and so qualify) have been researched and discussed by, among others, the GNC (1976), MacGuire (1969), Owen and Feldhusen (1970) and Singh and Smith (1975). In general, previous educational attainment and intelligence are both good predictors of success. However, it would appear that a basic intellectual level is essential for nursing, but any increase beyond that does not increase the likelihood of a trainee passing final examinations and thus succeeding in nurse training.

Thus, the implication is that intellectual capacity is only a partial predictor of success, and that there are other characteristics pertaining to the individual which correlate with, and are necessary for, completion of nurse training. One may then ask what these characteristics which are likely to be involved are, i.e. what 'sort of person' will succeed in nurse training? Suggestions include temperamental suitability, attitudes and motivation, which are non-cognitive factors which relate to personality.

Personality Assessment Among Nurses

The first reported research involving personality assessment among nurses in the UK was that of Petrie and Powell (1951) and Lee (1959) who, in trying to improve selection procedures for trainee nurses, hypothesised that personality was at least as important as intelligence in a good nurse. Since this work, numerous empirical studies have used personality measures (sometimes together with tests of intellectual and academic performance) among nurses, in particular trainee nurses.

A review of all the available research reports and papers (see Lewis and Cooper, 1976) found significant variation between references, which makes comparisons somewhat difficult, with regard to four main aspects of the studies. Firstly, there are variations with respect to sample design in terms of socio-economic and cultural factors, type of training programme, and sample size — several studies have been based on very small groups, which presents problems with the validity and interpretation of subsequent statistical analyses. Secondly, with regard to time of testing: the stage in nurse training at which personality testing takes place affects the data collected, the discussion and interpretation of information obtained from subsequent analysis, and any conclusions drawn. The later in training that the testing takes place, the greater will be the wastage that has taken place already, and the closer one will come to having measured the personality of 'stayers' or successful nurses only, rather than that of all trainees including those who will fail to complete their training.

Thirdly, there are differing objectives and methodology. Some work has been descriptive and focused on using personality tests to develop profiles of groups of trainee nurses, and has included comparisons between those who complete a nurse training programme and those who do not: other, predictive, research has been concerned with measure of success in nursing. The fourth differentiating aspect is the personality tests themselves. Those reported in the literature are many and include personality inventories and also projective tests, and measure a wide range of personality traits, both behavioural and pathological. Further, most were developed in the USA and so present some problems of transference and comparability when used in the UK.

The review of Lewis and Cooper showed that previous researchers had found some differences between personality profiles for trainee nurses and normal populations, and between completing and non-completing trainees, and evidence (albeit limited) of the ability of personality measurements to predict completion of a nurse training programme. However, the empirical work in Britain has proved, to some extent, disappointing in so far as six of the nine projects reviewed included relatively small samples, five were primarily concerned with psychiatric trainees and one with experimental course students, and four used somewhat obscure personality assessment measures (see Table 1.1). Consequently, none of them focused on a large sample of nurses in general training using a well-known and validated test to measure behavioural personality traits. Additionally, several of the British studies have considered either only starting trainees, or 'stayers' (after one year, 18 months, etc.) as compared with leavers. Less attention, by three researchers only, has been given to finishing/successful trainees, and subsequent comparisons between completing and non-completing students and pupils.

Thus, it seemed that there was a need and opportunity for further personality measurement among trainee nurses in the UK, to try to identify personality profiles of nurses who survive training programmes, which could be used in the development of future recruitment and selection criteria for nursing — based in part on personality — with a view to reducing wastage from nurse training[1].

Fieldwork

The research at UMIST involved data collection among newly recruited student and pupil nurses in general training (n = 895) in nine schools of nursing in England and Wales. A further group of nurses (n = 69) comprised mental illness and mental subnormality trainees in one health area. All nurses starting their training during a twelve month period in each school (1976/77) were seen during their introductory training course, when they completed a substantive survey questionnaire and Cattell's 16PF personality test (1963), the total sample being 964 learners.

Twelve months was considered to be an appropriate period to study, as one year will take account of differences between intakes within a school with regard to age and marital status, i.e. the sample for each school was representative of the intakes for that school. However, one year is also a sufficiently short period for any changes in the economic climate, which could affect reasons for entry to nurse training and the effectiveness of the various recruitment activities, to be of minimal importance.

The survey questionnaire was designed to determine the characteristics of a 'typical' sample of trainees with regard to their socio-economic and educational background, to discover their reasons for entering nursing, and to assess the relative importance of numerous sources of

Table 1.1: British personality studies

Author	Sample		Tests/Assessment	Objectives
Birch (1975)	85 students 51 pupils	all female, in general training	16PF + others	To compare students with pupils To compare leavers with stayers (at end of one year)
Brown and Stones (1972)	404 male psychiatric students		Eysenck Pers. Inventory + Tutors Assessment	To compare students with norms To compare leavers with stayers
Burton (1972)	66 psychiatric students		16PF + Tutors' Ratings	To compare successful with unsuccessful students (i.e. completing or not)
Caine (1964)	16 general nurses 20 general trainees 16 mental nurses 19 mental trainees		Kuder Preference Record	To compare trainees with norms To compare trainees with trained nurses To compare mental with general nurses
Cordiner (1968)	303 general students 19 psychiatric students (294F and 25M)		16PF + Tutors' Ratings	To compare students with US norms
Cordiner and Hall (1971)	192 female students		Motivational Analysis Test	To compare students with US norms To compare completing with non-completing students
Grygier (1957)	14 female 7 male	psychiatric trainees	Dynamic Pers. Inventory + Tutors' Ratings	To compare DPI with Tutor Ratings
Reaveley and Wilson (1972)	30 female 31 male	psychiatric students	16PF + other tests	To compare men with women To compare leavers with stayers
Singh (1971) and Singh and Smith (1975)	229 students on experimental courses 625 other SRN students		16PF + AVL + other tests	To compare experimental students with other SRN students To compare experimental students with US norms To compare completing with non-completing students

information and communications about nursing. Cattell's 16PF personality test was chosen as it is a well-known and a widely validated personality test, designed to measure behavioural personality traits. Further, it is perhaps the most comprehensive of all single personality tests in its coverage of personality dimensions with the primary sources traits, representing the basic variables in the total personality structure of an individual, and British editions of the test were available. Form C of the 16PF was used, comprising 105 three-alternative choice items from which raw scores are produced for each of the 16 personality source traits — descriptions of which are presented in Table 1.2.

Table 1.2: Primary factors of the 16PF

Low Score Description	Source Trait	High Score Description
Reserved (Sizothymia) detached, critical, aloof	A	**Outgoing** (Affectothymia) easy-going, warmhearted, participating
Less Intelligent (Lower scholastic mental capacity) concrete-thinking	B	**More Intelligent** (Higher scholastic mental capacity) bright, abstract thinking
Affected by Feelings (Lower ego strength) emotionally less stable	C	**Emotionally Stable** (Higher ego strength) calm, mature, faces reality
Humble (Submissive) mild, accommodating, easily led, docile, conforming, obedient	E	**Assertive** (Dominance) aggressive, stubborn, competitive
Sober (Desurgency) prudent, serious, taciturn	F	**Happy-go-lucky** (Surgency) gay, impulsively lively, enthusiastic
Expedient (Weaker superego strength) disregards rules, feels few obligations	G	**Conscientious** (Stronger superego strength) persevering, staid, moralistic, rule-bound
Shy (Threctia) restrained, timid, threat-sensitive	H	**Venturesome** (Parmia) socially bold, uninhibited, spontaneous
Tough-minded (Harria) realistic, self-reliant, no nonsense	I	**Tender-minded** (Premsia) clinging, over-protected, sensitive, dependent
Trusting (Alaxia) adaptable, free of jealousy, easy to get along with, accepting conditions	L	**Suspicious** (Protension) self-opinionated, jealous, hard to fool
Practical (Praxernia) careful, down to earth concerns, proper, regulated by external realities, conventional	M	**Imaginative** (Autia) wrapped up in inner urgencies, careless of practical matters, bohemian
Forthright (Artlessness) natural, artless, pretentious, genuine but socially clumsy	N	**Shrewd** (Shrewdness) calculating, wordly, astute, penetrating, polished, socially aware
Self-assured (Untroubled adequacy) confident, serene, complacent, placid	O	**Apprehensive** (Guilt proneness) self-reproaching, worrying, troubled, insecure
Conservative (Conservatism) respecting established ideas, tolerant of traditional difficulties	Q1	**Experimenting** (Radicalism) liberal, free-thinking, analytical
Group-dependent (Group adherence) a joiner and a sound follower	Q2	**Self-sufficient** (Self-sufficiency) resourceful, prefers own decisions
Undisciplined self-conflict (Low integration) self-conflict, follows own urges, careless of protocol/social rules	Q3	**Controlled** (High self-concept control) socially precise, exacting will power, following self-image, compulsive
Relaxed (low ergic tension) tranquil, unfrustrated, composed	Q4	**Tense** (high ergic tension) fretful, frustrated, driven, overwrought

Results

Forty-eight per cent of the participating learners were SRN trainees and 42 per cent were SEN trainees, being 4 per cent of all student and pupil entrants to general training in England and Wales in 1976/77. Ninety-two per cent of all respondents were female and 82 per cent single: further, 62 per cent were aged 18-19 years, 20 per cent aged 20-23 years and 18 per cent were 24 years or older. The students were younger than pupils and less likely to be married, as were women as compared with men: the relative proportions being in line with aggregate GNC data.

Educational Background

The nursing schools all specified certain minimum academic entry standards, in terms of GCEs/CSEs and/or the D test, but in practice their entrants were more highly qualified — as a result of the high demand for places in nurse training. 72.2 per cent of all respondents had passed GCE 'O' levels at school or in college (52 per cent having been to some institute of further education) and 57.7 per cent had CSE examination passes[2], students having more passes than pupils (p < .01). 53 per cent of respondents had achieved their GCE/CSE successes in one year, 39 per cent took two years and 8 per cent needed more time. Additional information showed that 44 per cent possessed 'other qualifications, certificates or diplomas', of whom 26 per cent had one or more 'A' levels or above — several had been to university or teacher training college, and 19 per cent had other academic qualifications. These percentages were significantly higher (p < .01), as one might expect, for students than for pupils.

More detailed analysis of learners in general training only showed that as many as 37 per cent of students had 3 or fewer 'O' levels — comprising mainly mature students, and that 15 per cent of pupils had 4 or more 'O' levels — which would make them strong candidates for student training in many nursing schools (see Table 1.3). When these findings are compared with appropriate GNC data for all students and pupils in general training in the nine survey schools and in England and Wales as a whole, it may be seen that the responding students are typical of their training school but have less 'O' levels than the 'average' student. However, the pupils in the survey were neither typical of their training school nor of all pupils, possibly because GCE grade 1 had been included as a GCE 'O' level pass.

Table 1.3: GCE 'O' level examination passes (general training)

Sample Group	O passes %	1-3 %	4-6 %	≥7 passes %
Students				
Survey (n = 461)	13.2	23.9	42.1	20.8
9 schools of nursing	30.2	7.7	38.4	23.7
All England and Wales*	20.7	6.8	38.6	33.9
Pupils				
Survey (n = 406)	44.3	41.1	13.8	0.8
9 schools of nursing	86.5	4.8	6.8	1.9
All England and Wales	80.4	7.1	10.6	1.9

* (GNC for England and Wales, 15 December 1977)

Correlates of Success in Nurse Training

Follow-up information was received over a three-year period from the participating schools of nursing, which enabled the trainees' progress to be monitored, and analysis of 'wastage' from training programmes with regard to time of leaving, reasons for withdrawal from training, and correlates of success and failure in nurse training. Findings presented in this context pertain to 320 students (224 of whom completed their training and passed their examinations, and 96 withdrew from training) and 389 pupils (282 of whom completed, with 107 leaving training), all of whom were females in general training.

Subsequent analysis showed completing students and pupils to be younger, and more likely to be single, than those who failed to complete training programmes ($p < .01$ in each case). The mature student or pupil seemed to have more difficulty in completing her training programme, possibly as a result of marriage or family responsibilities; e.g. a number of older, married, trainees appeared to have family commitments which were not compatible with the rigours of nurse training.

Further, 58 per cent of completing students had at least 5 GCE 'O' levels as compared with 46 per cent of leavers, and 55 per cent of stayers had some CSE passes as compared with 44 per cent of leavers (both significant differences, $p < .05$). Similarly, completing pupils were more likely than leavers to have 'O' levels, and 69 per cent of successful pupils had CSEs as compared with 47 per cent of leavers (a significant difference, $p < .01$). Additionally, successful pupils were more likely than unsuccessful ones to have had some prior experience of further education and a shorter gap between school/further education and nurse training. This would seem to suggest that trainees who have been away from the educational sector for some time find it more difficult to adjust to the nurse training school environment.

These findings parallel those from earlier research which show previous educational attainment to be a good predictor of success in nurse training, although the educational entry standards in the participating schools were such that most entering trainees had more than the minimum requirements and so would not be expected to be struggling academically.

Personality Testing Among Trainee Nurses

The total sample of 964 trainees had to be subdivided for analysis of personality variables: firstly, as men and women must be considered separately; and secondly, as a number of training courses were represented which may attract differing personality types, i.e. student/ pupils training, and general/mental illness/mental subnormality training. Subsequently *t* tests were used to compare mean scores between the various groups of female and male trainees.

Differences between Training Courses, and Sexes

Data for female trainees showed that the students in general training were more intelligent than their pupil counterparts (factor B, $p < .01$), but had a lower mean score on factor G ($p < .01$), i.e. they were less conscientious and rule-bound. Girls on mental illness/subnormality courses had higher scores than both general students and pupils on factor M ($p < .01$): they were more imaginative, unconventional and unconcerned with everyday matters.

For male trainees, three main differences were apparent. General students had more disregard for rules and regulations (factor G, $p < .01$), were more self-opinionated and suspicious (factor L, $p < .01$), and were more experienced, hard-headed and analytical (factor N, $p < .01$) than either general pupils or mental illness/subnormality trainees. Further, there were a number of differences between male and female general students, and between male and female general pupils – as one might expect. However, the personality profiles for male and female mental illness/subnormality trainees were remarkably similar, i.e. no differences at the 1 per cent level.

Comparison of Trainee Nurse Groups with Normal Populations and Previously Tested Groups of Trainee Nurses

Further meaning is added to the interpretation of personality test data by comparison with some normal population and/or previously tested group(s). In the present research the personality scores for students and pupils in general training were compared with data from a sample of 2584 university undergraduates (see Saville and Blinkorn, 1976), and with personality data available from research by Singh (NFER TIS/05.05; Nursing Times, 1971) – in particular that for 625 trainees on traditional SRN courses.

The resulting *t*-test values showed differences (p < .01) between the female students and pupils in general training and Singh's students for as many as 11 of the 16 personality factors. This must surely represent a combination of the use of different editions of the test form (i.e. Singh used an early American edition of the 16PF), testing conditions, and the nature of the samples -- Singh's students were certainly not typical of all student nurses in general training. There was also variation (p < .01) between the female students and pupils in general training and Saville and Blinkorn's female undergraduates for most of the factors. Consideration of all the information pertaining to females indicated three personality factors of particular interest: F, O and Q1. For factor F, there were no differences between the various nurse groups, but the university undergraduates had lower scores, i.e. they were more serious and restrained. *t*-test values for factor O provided evidence that Singh's nurses were more confident and self-assured than either of the other nurse groups or the university undergraduates. On factor Q1, the undergraduates were found to be more experimenting and interested in intellectual matters than the survey nurses, who in turn had higher scores than Singh's nurses – who seemed to be more conservative and inclined to go along with tradition.

Analysis for males provided evidence of similar personality profiles for general nurse trainees and university undergraduates. However, the student nurses had a lower mean intelligence score (factor B) than the undergraduates (p < .01), and the pupil nurses differed from the undergraduates (p < .01) on two factors (G+, N-), which are consistent with the differences between male students and pupils in general training already highlighted.

Comparisons between Completing and Non-completing Trainee Nurses

A most interesting and valuable section of the analysis was the investigation of possible differences in personality characteristics between completing and non-completing trainees. This was carried out with a view to trying to identify personality profiles of nurses who survive training programmes and pass their final examinations, which in turn could have use in the development of future selection criteria for nursing.

The four major relevant groups, i.e. completing and non-completing students and pupils in general training (all female), were investigated using, once again, *t*-test analysis to consider possible differences between sample groups. There was little variation between the two student groups; however consideration of completing and non-completing pupils highlighted several significant differences.

The completing pupils were more venturesome and socially bold (H+), i.e. they were ready to try new things and were able to face wear and tear, in dealing with people and gruelling emotional situations, without fatigue. They were also more self-confident and self-assured (O-), i.e. having a mature, non-anxious confidence in themselves and a capacity to deal with things: such people are also characterised by resistance and unshakeable nerve. Finally, the completing pupils would seem to be more group-dependent (Q2-), i.e. preferring to work and make decisions with other people, but also dependent on social approval and admiration.

In contrast, the pupils who wasted from training had lower scores on factor H: they were shy, restrained and retiring, possibly with inferiority feelings and a tendency to be slow in expressing themselves. People with low H scores are often seen as disliking occupations with personal contacts, and are not given to keeping in contact with all that is going on around them. This group also had high factor O scores, which implies they were apprehensive and worrying, and perhaps moody — such people do not usually feel accepted in groups or feel free to participate. Finally, the leavers had higher scores than stayers on factor Q2, which suggests a degree of temperamental independence, accustomed to doing things their way, and making decisions and acting on their own. These differences between completing and non-completing pupils appear to be consistent with each other, and also with general preconceptions of what is expected of a successful (trainee) nurse. Thus, it would seem that high scores on factors O and Q2, and low scores on factor H, might imply an element of 'unsuitability' for nurse training.

The Newly Qualified Nurse and the Completing Trainee Nurse

Findings from the personality assessment carried out among samples of qualified nurses at various stages in their careers, i.e. at a number of levels of seniority and with differing lengths of service, are discussed elsewhere (e.g. Cooper *et al.*, 1976; Lewis, 1980). However, two of the groups researched were newly registered nurses and newly enrolled nurses, and their personality assessments are considered in this final section, together with those for completing trainee nurses. Almost all completing trainees do register or enrol and continue nursing, if only for some minimum period of time, and consequently there should be no differences between the personality profiles for completing trainees (assessed at the start of their training) and for newly registered/enrolled nurses. To prove this hypothesis would also be a measure of consistency of the personality test itself.

The personality test scores for completing students (n = 224) from the participating nursing schools were compared with those for newly registered nurses (n = 47), and the scores for completing pupils (n = 282) compared with those for newly enrolled nurses (n = 105). Once again, all were females in general nursing.

Only one difference was found between completing students and newly registered nurses, on factor G (p < .05): the newly-registered nurses would seem to be more conscientious and persevering than the completing students. However, there were — perhaps surprisingly — three differences between completing pupils and newly enrolled nurses. The completing pupils had higher mean scores (p<.05) than the newly enrolled nurses on factor B (intelligence) and factor F — the completing pupils would appear to be somewhat more happy-go-lucky and impulsive than the newly-enrolled nurses, who seemed to be more sober and serious. The third difference was for factor Q2: here, completing pupils would seem to be more in need of group support than newly-enrolled nurses. These differences might, however, be attributable, in part, to some personality change, i.e. the variation between personality scores for a girl in her introductory training course and for an older, qualified and more experienced woman.

Summary

In this chapter the assessment of a number of intellectual and personality characteristics of trainee nurses has been described, data having been collected from a total of 964 learners as they began their nurse training programmes. Discussion has centred on both the intellectual and personality profiles of the participating learners, and some correlates of success in and wastage from nurse training — based on statistical comparisons between completing and non-completing students and pupils in general training. The findings, together with others from the same research investigation (see Lewis, 1979), have relevance for the development of future recruitment and selection procedures designed to reduce wastage from nurse training and from the nursing profession, i.e. to recruit and select trainees who will not only qualify as nurses but also see nursing as a long-term career and remain actively involved in the nursing profession.

Data collection was focused on assessment of the participating trainees using elements from a structured questionnaire together with an objective psychometric test. A variety of other individual charac- teristics and perceptions of trainee nurses are considered in subsequent chapters in this section, with research methodologies comprising a number of techniques to include objective tests, interviews and self- assessment methods.

Notes

1. However, ability to complete a nurse training programme and become registered or enrolled is a myopic view of success in nursing. A number of quali- fying nurses, for whom completion may merely be a reflection of the desire to secure a qualification, will leave at the first possible opportunity, and many others will stay in the profession for only a few years. Real success in nursing may be better defined in terms of the person qualifying as a nurse who feels that he or she has entered a life-time profession and who will remain actively involved in nursing.

Thus, one can ask whether personality profiles of qualified nurses, at various stages in their careers, are similar to, or different from, the profiles of successful trainees. If profiles do differ, then one would want to generate personality-based selection criteria from samples of nurses who have been actively involved in nursing for some time, and who have achieved some measure of success within the profession, rather than selecting trainees based on criteria validated on students who have just completed a training programme. Consequently, further aspects of research at UMIST, reported elsewhere, have centred on personality assessment among groups of qualified nurses to try to establish realistic personality-based criteria of 'suitability' for nursing.

2. CSE grade 1 (where specified) was included as 'O' level, and subjects named at both GCE and CSE were included only as GCE passes.

References

Barr, A. (1959) 'Training of student nurses', *British Journal of Preventive and Social Medicine, 13*(3), 149-55

Birch, J.A. (1975) *To Nurse or Not to Nurse*, Royal College of Nursing, London

Brown, R.G.S. (1974) 'After registration: patterns of success and wastage,' *Nursing Times, 70*, 58-61, 89-91

Brown, R.G.S. (1974) 'The enrolled nurse: male nurses', *Nursing Times, 70*, 125-8

Brown, R.G.S. and Stones, R.W.H. (1972) 'Personality and intelligence characteristics of male nurses,' *International Journal of Nursing Studies, 9*(3), 167-77

Burton, D.A. (1972) 'The selection of nurses by discriminant analysis,' *International Journal of Nursing Studies, 9*(2), 77-84

Caine, T.M. (1964) 'Personality tests for nurses,' *Nursing Times, 60*, 973-4

Cattell, R.B. (1963) 'The sixteen personality factor questionnaire (the 16PF)', Institute of Personality and Ability Testing, Illinois

Cooper, C.L., Lewis, B.R. and Moores, B. (1976) 'Personality profiles of long serving senior nurses: implications for recruitment and selection,' *International Journal of Nursing Studies, 13*, 251-7

Cordiner, C.M. (1968) 'Personality testing of Aberdeen student nurses,' *Nursing Times, 64*(6), 178-80

Cordiner, C.M. and Hall, D.J. (1971) 'The use of the motivational analysis test in the selection of Scottish nursing students,' *Nursing Research, 20*(4), 356-62

Cross, K.W. and Hall, D.L.A. (1954) 'Survey of entrants to nurse training schools and of student nurse wastage in the Birmingham Region,' *British Journal of Preventive and Social Medicine, 8*(2), 70-6

General Nursing Council for England and Wales (1966) *Student Nurse Wastage*

General Nursing Council for England and Wales (1976) The Student and Pupil Nurse Population: January 1976 (unpublished)

Grygier, P. (1957) 'Personality and the selection of nurses,' *Nursing Times, 53*, 910-12

Lee, T. (1959) 'The selection of student nurses: a revised procedure,' *Occupational Psychology, 33*(4), 209-15

Lewis, B.R. and Cooper, C.L. (1976) 'Personality measurement among nurses: a review,' *International Journal of Nursing Studies, 13*, 209-29

Lewis, B.R. (1977) 'Marketing of nursing as a career,' *European Journal of Marketing, 11*(6), 432-44

Lewis, B.R. The Marketing of Nursing, unpublished Ph.D. Thesis, Department of Management Sciences, UMIST, 1979

Lewis, B.R. (1980) 'Personality profiles for qualified nurses: possible implications for recruitment and selection of trainne nurses,' *International Journal of Nursing Studies, 17*, 221-34

MacGuire, J.M. (1969) *Threshold to Nursing*, Occasional Papers on Social Administration, No. 30, Bell, London

Owen, S.V. and Feldhusen, J.F. (1970) 'Effectiveness of three models of multivariate prediction of academic success in nursing education,' *Nursing Research, 19*(6), 517-25

Petrie, A. and Powell, M.B. (1951) 'The selection of student nurses in England,' *Journal of Applied Psychology, 35*(4), 281-6

Reaveley, W. and Wilson, L.J. (1972) 'Personality structure of general and psychiatric student nurses: a comparison,' *International Journal of Nursing Studies, 9*(4), 225-34

Revans, R.W. (1964) *Standards for Morale: Cause and Effect in Hospitals*, Nuffield Provincial Hospitals Trust, Oxford University Press, Oxford

Saville, P. and Blinkorn, S. (1976) *Undergraduate Personality by Factored Scales*, NFER Publishing Co. Ltd., Windsor, Berks

Singh, A. (1971) 'The student nurse on experimental courses,' *International Journal of Nursing Studies, 8*, 189-205, 207-18

Singh, A. (1971) 'Norms for first year student nurses: general intelligence and personality,' *Nursing Times, 67*, 117-20

Singh, A. (1956) *The 16PF Questionnaire, American Edition, Form C: Norms for First Year Student Nurses*, NFER Publishing Co. Ltd., Windsor, Berks

Singh, A. and Smith, J. (1975) 'Retention and withdrawal of student nurses,' *International Journal of Nursing Studies, 12*, 43-56

Thompson, A.G.H. (1974) An Attitudinal Analysis of Student Nurse Morale, and Correlation with Wastage, unpublished B.Sc. Dissertation, Department of Management Sciences, UMIST, 1974

2 ANXIETY AND CONFLICT IN NURSE EDUCATION

John A. Birch

The volume of literature on stress and the many and varied topics falling under this rubric is vast indeed. Lazarus (1966) pointed out that if this huge literature should be removed or abandoned by scientists, 'devastating effect on the volume of physiological research and writing would result'. In an attempt to explain the reason for such a voluminous activity, he states: 'stress is a universal human and animal phenomenon resulting in intense and distressing experience and appears to be a tremendous influence in behaviour'.

Hilgarde (1966), in writing the foreword to Levitt's work *The Psychology of Anxiety*, expressed the view that we are living in an age of anxiety, the causes of which lie variously between war, mobility of people resulting in disturbance of 'rootedness', uncertainty about child-rearing practice, moral standards and doubts in the religious field. He states, 'whatever the cause, the signs of anxiety lie around us in part through social disaffection and delinquency, alienation and anomy, alcoholism, drug addiction, divorce and mental illness'.

My previous research (Birch, 1975) led me to speculate on whether anxiety *per se* was a significant influence in withdrawal of students from schools of nursing. Revans (1964) had described hospitals as 'institutions cradled in anxiety'. Menzies (1961) investigated ways in which nursing administration attempted to reduce anxiety in nurses, but effectively increased the level in the attempt. The editorial of the *Nursing Mirror* of 24 March 1977 states,

> Almost from the day she enters training, the student nurse is plunged into a moral dilemma of a magnitude that would tax the conscience of one much more advanced in years, wisdom and experience. Yet to fulfil her duties towards her patients properly, the nurse must learn to face situations which present agonisingly difficult choices of action, and trust conscience to be her guide.

It was the Briggs Report, however, that inspired my research into measurable anxiety levels in nursing learners. Whilst the Report of the

Committee of Nursing is for the majority a mandate for new Statutory Bodies, modules of training and Colleges of Nursing and Midwifery, for me it is a shrewd textbook of educational philosophy with profound insights into anxiety as experienced by learners. Careful reading of the Report will reveal many specific comments on anxiety, such as, 'We have been struck by the power of the pressures on the trainee nurse . . . given the highly demanding work and the profound and often unpredictable stresses . . .'

The present study set out to measure anxiety levels of students and pupils nurses (n = 207) in the first two years of hospital experience as it arises, because of experiences in the clinical situation and as a result of the curriculum planned by the tutorial staff in block periods of study. In addition, it was planned to measure conflict in terms of healthy and unhealthy thinking. The sample was taken from four schools of nursing in the North of England. The design included the use of the following instruments.

(1)   *The IPAT Anxiety Scale (Self-analysis Form)*
      (R.B. Cattell and I.H. Scheier, 1963)

The IPAT Anxiety Scale (otherwise named the Self-analysis Form) was devised in 1957 as a 'brief, non-stressful, clinically-valid questionnaire for measuring anxiety'.

By factor analysis, the IPAC investigators identified sixteen personality traits, as measured in the 16PF Personality Test. Five of these 16 dimensions involve questions which 'look like' anxiety, and 'cluster', indicating that they are related to each other statistically to a significant degree. Cattell's five oblique first order factors are Q3(-) Defective integration, Lack of self sentiment, C(-) Ego weakness, lack of ego strength, L Suspiciousness or Paranoid pressure. These first-order factors intercorrelate to define Cattell's second-order factor U.I. 24 described as 'a single unitary index best equipped to represent *the* anxiety factor.'

Cattell suggests that a sten[1] of 1, 2 or 3 indicates stability, security and mental health. Stens 4, 5, 6 and 7 are still in the normal range but those with a sten of 7 should be seen as borderline high anxiety and warrant careful follow up. Stens of 8, 9 and 10 suggest 'definite psychological morbidity, almost certain to have an adverse effect on work and social/emotional adjustment of the individual.'

(2)   *The Rotter Incomplete Sentences Blank* (College Form)
       (Julian B. Rotter, 1950)

This semi-structured projective test 'allows the subject wide latitude in expressing conflicts, thoughts and fantasies, and usually produces a wealth of emotionally toned material.'

Rotter (1950) has successfully described a method of rationally derived quantitative scoring which brings the use of the instruments into the reach of persons not qualified in the field of clinical psychology, for example, tutors, counsellors, etc. The specimen responses contained in the manual are comprehensive and numerous, providing a basis for the researcher to develop considerable expertise given a little practice. In the present research, the author's standard form was used without modification, as in my previous investigation. The given items range over questions of considerable interest to nurse educators and individual responses can be treated at a 'common sense' level without attempting a clinical evaluation. This was the most successful at the projective tests used in Kelly and Fiske's research (1951) on selecting clinical psychologists.

(3)   *Self-devised Anxiety Area Questionnaire*

In order to identify specific areas of anxiety existing in the daily routine of the nurses in the sample, it was first necessary to list items which by their nature might produce anxiety. These items were assembled after considerable conversation with nurses in training. Included in the list are factors discovered almost accidentally in my previous research. The items finally decided upon ranged from dealing with patients' bodily discharges to care of the dying, relationships with members of the multi-disciplinary team and controversial issues like cardiac arrest and its treatment. Interspersed among the factors are a few items relating to hospital administration and personal fears of nursing staff, for example, 'fear of growing old' and 'fear of the dark'. A five-point scale was devised in an attempt to measure expressed anxiety, the headings being: very great stress, great stress, some stress, very little stress and no stress. The questionnaire was offered to the examinees and the following instructions given verbally and in writing, 'Please indicate the degree of stress you have experienced as you have come to terms with your work on the wards. Stress should be taken to mean your feelings of anxiety in a given situation.'

Methodology

Students and pupils were tested on the IPAT Anxiety Scale during the introductory courses and at eight-monthly intervals thereafter. The Self-devised Anxiety Questionnaire was administered at eight months and two years after commencement of training. It was hypothesised that as nurse training proceeded, levels of anxiety, as measured by both of these tests, should diminish with experience. The Rotter Incomplete Sentences Blank was completed during the introductory course.

The block timetable of each student and pupil was analysed, principally to attempt to discover the degree of emphasis placed on psychological theory, as it was felt that the degree of stress experienced might be directly related to the lack of preparation in the behavioural sciences. The main hypothesis states that 'The pattern of general nurse education produces anxiety in the student and pupil because of its failure to prepare the student and pupil adequately for his/her role in relation to the patient's psychological needs.'

Following this analysis, a structured interview was carried out with each learner to discover how specific areas of practice, shown by the self-devised test to be productive of anxiety, were supported theoretically. The identical questionnaire was given to a sample of tutorial staff in the appropriate training schools.

Analysis of Results

Levels of Anxiety on IPAT Scale

Pupils demonstrated greater anxiety than students throughout their entire training ($p < 0.05$). It is interesting to note the percentage of learners who scored at the 7th sten and above. During the introductory course, 90 of the 207 people in the sample scored at the 7th sten and above (43.48 per cent), 48 at the 8th sten, 24 at the 9th sten and two at the 10th sten.

At tests two, three and four over the first two years of training, the percentage of learners scoring at the 7th sten and above continued to be relatively high, being 30.39, 29.76 and 36.48 per cent respectively. 33.9 per cent of all learners scored at the 8th sten after two years, 13.84 per cent at the 9th sten and 3.72 per cent at the 10th sten.

A chi-square test was applied to the four test results, comparing those who scored at the 7th sten and above. Between test one and test two there was a highly significant drop in anxiety ($p < 0.00001$), but when test one was compared with test four, there was no significant difference in anxiety levels. Thus the anxiety level in the introductory course, after reducing at eight months and 16 months, regained its high level after two years, perhaps in part because the pupils in the sample were facing their final examinations at the time.

Franklin (1974) tested 160 male patients about to undergo major surgery, using the IPAT Anxiety Scale. The percentage of patients scoring at the 7th sten and above was compared with the present sample at all points of training. In the introductory course, the percentage of learners scoring at this level was no different from Franklin's anxious surgical patients, who scored significantly higher than the general population; that is to say, while in the introductory course the nurses were as anxious as the patients. After eight months, the nurses scored significantly lower than the patients ($p < 0.0001$). After 16 months, however, the learner anxiety was again equal to that of the patients, and after two years of training, the level of learner anxiety was significantly greater than in the patients ($p < 0.05$) (Table 2.1).

Table 2.1: Percentage reaching the 7th sten or above at test one, two, three and four for pupils and students, together, compared with Franklin's surgical admissions

	Introductory Course		8 months		16 months		24 months		Franklin's Patients	
	Test 1		Test 2		Test 3		Test 4		On Admission	
	No.	%	No.	%	No.	%	No.	%	No.	%
7th sten	90	43.48	55	30.99	50	29.76	58	36.48	66	41.25
8th sten	48	23.10	26	14.36	33	19.64	38	33.90	24	15.00
9th sten	24	11.60	7	3.87	22	13.09	22	13.84	17	10.62
10th sten	2	0.97	–	–	7	4.17	6	3.72	3	1.88

Levels of Conflict on Rotter Incomplete Sentences Blank

Reference to Table 2.2 will indicate that there was no significant statistical difference between the scores of students and pupils in the introductory course. A mean score of 123.46 and 124.67 was achieved by students and pupils respectively.

What the analysis did unequivocally show, however, was a highly significant difference between both student and pupil stayers and leavers. (The stayer is defined as a learner who remains in training for the period of research, i.e. for the first two years of student nurse training and the complete course of two years for pupil nurse training.)

Significantly more student leavers (53 per cent) than student stayers (15 per cent) scored more than 135 (p<0.01) and significantly more pupil leavers (43 per cent) than pupil stayers (17 per cent) had a score greater than 135 (p<0.01). As my previous research (Birch, 1975) had shown a 2 per cent level of significant difference between all stayers and all leavers, this further evident difference between the two groups in question (student and pupil stayers and leavers) adds to the attractive proposition that the instrument would be useful in the selection process of students and pupils at the stage of application. For selection purposes, 53 per cent of student leavers and 43 per cent of pupil leavers would immediately be identified. If, however, the cut-off point of 143 be invoked as in my previous research, 41.3 per cent of student leavers (seven persons) and 38.2 per cent of pupil leavers (eight persons) would be identified. Only 4.26 per cent of student stayers (three persons) and 5.6 per cent of pupil stayers (four persons) scored above this point. It could be argued, therefore, that if the instrument had been used as an absolute screening device, a reasonable percentage of potential dropouts would have been excluded and seven persons denied training, who, as it happens, have succeeded until at least the end of the second year of training.

Analysis of Self-devised Questionnaire

The stress questionnaire, containing 56 items of professional experience likely to cause anxiety, was but a subjective expression of those areas needing specific educational application in the curriculum of nurse training. It was a method of encouraging students and pupils to identify aspects of experience which in their opinion were anxiety provoking, and also to relate the findings of this questionnaire to an analysis of the timetable prepared for learners during block periods of study in order to indicate the degree to which both learners and their tutors considered behavioural aspects of care to have been adequately considered.

The questionnaires, completed at eight and 24 months, showed that the first 25 items causing stress had not changed significantly. Some confidence can be placed in the questionnaire, therefore, in truly indicating those areas which need to receive special emphasis in curriculum planning. Table 2.3 shows the rank order into which items fall.

Table 2.2: Distribution of Rotter Incomplete Sentences Blank scores for students and pupils, and student and pupil stayers and leavers

Score	Students		Pupils		Student Stayers		Student Leavers		Pupil Stayers		Pupil Leavers	
	No.	Cum. %	No.	Cum. %	No.	Cum. %	No.	Cum. %	No.	Cum. %	No.	Cum %
180-183	–	–	1	100	–	–	–	–	–	–	1	100
176-179	–	–	--	–	--	–	–	–	–	–	–	–
172-175	–	–	–	–	–	–	–	–	–	–	–	–
168-171	2	100	2	97.8	–	–	2	100	–	–	2	95.2
164-167	–	–	–	–	–	–	–	–	–	–	–	–
160-163	2	97.8	–	–	1	100	1	88.2	–	–	–	–
156-159	–	–	2	95.6	–	–	–	–	1	100	1	85.7
152-155	2	95.6	1	94.5	–	–	2	82.3	1	98.6	–	–
148-151	1	94.5	4	90.2	1	98.6	–	–	1	97.2	3	80.9
144-147	3	90.2	2	88.0	1	97.2	2	70.5	1	95.8	1	66.6
140-143	7	83.5	3	84.7	7	87.7	–	–	2	94.4	1	61.8
136-139	3	80.2	7	77.1	1	86.3	2	58.7	6	91.6	1	57.0
132-135	3	76.9	3	73.8	3	82.2	–	–	2	83.1	1	52.2
128-131	11	64.8	4	69.5	8	71.4	3	46.9	3	80.3	1	47.4
124-127	11	52.7	12	56.5	10	57.9	1	29.3	8	76.1	4	42.6
120-123	8	43.9	12	43.5	7	48.4	1	23.4	10	64.8	2	23.6
116-119	9	34.0	10	32.6	9	36.2	–	–	10	50.7	–	–
112-115	7	26.3	13	18.5	6	28.1	1	17.5	12	36.6	1	14.1
108-111	8	17.5	7	10.9	8	17.3	–	–	6	19.7	1	9.3
104-107	4	13.1	4	6.6	4	11.9	–	–	3	11.2	1	4.5
100-103	5	7.6	2	4.4	3	7.8	2	5.7	2	7.0	–	–
96-99	1	6.5	1	3.3	1	6.4	–	–	1	4.2	–	–
92-95	1	5.4	1	2.2	1	5.0	–	–	1	2.8	–	–
88-91	3	2.1	1	1.1	3	0.9	–	–	1	1.4	–	–
	91		92		74		17		71		21	
mean	123.46		124.67		120.50		136.35		120.90		137.43	
	16.92		16.79		14.59		20.55		13.41		20.77	
variance	286.29		281.87		212.83		422.24		179.95		431.36	

	No significant difference	$(p < 0.01)$	$(p < 0.01)$

Table 2.3: Rank order of stress areas revealed in questionnaires
completed after eight and 24 months of training

Rank Order After Eight Months	Stress Area	Rank Order After 24 Months
1	Nursing of patients in great pain	3
2	Being shown up on the wards in front of patients and other staff	2
3	Progress tests in block periods of study	6
4	Dealing with patients with cancer	5
5	Care of the terminally ill	4
6	Care of the dying	6
7	Dealing with bereaved relatives	7
8	Changing wards	13
9	Your feelings of your own death	12
9	Your feelings of growing old	11
10	Understaffing	1
11	Last offices	8
12	Carrying out procedures before being taught in school	8
13	Late notification of off-duty	18
14	Dealing with sputum	11
15	Differing procedures in classroom and wards	19
16	Dealing with patients with cardiac arrest	10
17	Anticipation of night duty	16
18	Availability of study time	14
19	Dealing with nursing officers	20
19	Your feelings about being in the dark (literal darkness)	23
20	Your own progress report by ward sister	21
21	Dealing with doctors	25
22	Being left in charge of ward for short period, e.g. coffee break	24
23	Arrangements of social occasions	35
24	Dealing with bed sores	38
25	Dealing with patients on cardiac monitors	17
25	Dealing with ward sisters/charge nurses	34
26	Mopping up vomit	30
27	Dealing with the mentally disturbed	23
28	Dealing with relatives	26
29	Dealing with very old persons	31
29	Dealing with confused patients	37

Rank Order After Eight Months	Stress Area	Rank Order After 24 Months
30	Dealing with overdose cases	29
31	Writing of ward reports	26
31	Canteen facilities	28
32	Dealing with mutilated persons through casualty	31
33	Dealing with cases of colostomy/ileostomy	32
34	Dealing with tutors	36
35	Dealing with children with incurable diseases	9
36	Dealing with postoperative mastectomy	22
37	Dealing with incontinent patients	39
38	Disposing of faeces	40
38	Dealing with preoperative mastectomy	27
39	Dealing with staff nurses	41
40	The use of telephone communication	42
41	Dealing with patients of the opposite sex	43
42	Dealing with young female patients having abortions	33
43	Dealing with domestic staff	50
44	Dealing with out-patients on ward	47
45	Dealing with students/pupils a little senior to yourself	45
46	Dealing with SENs	44
47	Dealing with postoperative hysterectomy	46
48	Dealing with preoperative hysterectomy	48
49	Dealing with auxiliaries	49
50	Disposing of urine	51

Of the 28 areas causing the greatest amount of stress at eight months when set out in rank order, 20 assume a greater power, or remain the same, in their ability as stressors after 24 months.

It could be argued that at 24 months of training the stressors above should show a marked decline in their powers if professional education was effective in its ability to prepare students and pupils adequately. Rather the opposite appears to be the case and anxiety remains a striking factor of everyday occurrence.

Furthermore, there is a suggestion that it is largely within the behavioural aspects of care that the curriculum fails to reduce stress. It will be noted that the preponderance of stressors come within the broad category of death and dying.

Table 2.4: Areas increasing in stress power or significantly the same at 8 and 24 months

Behavioural	8 Months	24 Months
Nursing of patients in great pain	1	3
Being shown up on the wards in front of patients and other staff	2	2
Dealing with patients with cancer	4	5
Care of the terminally ill	5	4
Care of the dying	6	6
Dealing with bereaved relatives	7	7
Last offices	11	8
Dealing with cardiac arrest	16	10
Your feelings of your own death	9	12
Your feelings of growing old	9	11
Anticipating night duty	17	16
Your own progress report by ward sister	20	21
Dealing with patients on cardiac monitors	25	17
Administrative		
Understaffing	10	1
Carrying out procedures before being taught in school	12	15
Availability of study time	18	14
Dealing with nursing officers	19	20
Dealing with doctors	21	25
Being left in charge of ward for coffee breaks, etc.	22	24
Procedural		
Dealing with sputum	14	11

It is now time to begin to examine the curriculum, both by asking the learners about the content of the formal and informal education process, and by a direct analysis of the timetable as prepared by the tutorial staff.

Responses of Learners Compared with Tutors in Relation to the Curriculum

Death and Bereavement

Because of the learner's responsibility in taking the first initiative in the event of cardiac arrest, it was thought necessary to discover the extent to which the diagnosis of death features in the formal school timetable. The question was asked: 'Are the requirements for the diagnosis of death included formally in the school curriculum?' Seventeen per cent of pupils, 30 per cent of students and 35 per cent of tutorial staff answered 'yes'. Cardiac arrest ranks 16th at eight months and 10th at 24 months, out of 56 stress items. The considerable difference between training schools and the marked disadvantage that pupils experienced, except in school two where pupils fared better than students, can be seen in Table 2.5. School one placed pupils in an invidious position in that only 8 per cent answered 'yes'. Both learners and tutors were in agreement on this item, in that only 35 per cent of tutors admitted to including instruction in this vital area.

Table 2.5: Percentage answering 'yes' to the question: 'Are the requirements for the diagnosis of death included formally in the school curriculum?

School 1		School 2		School 3		School 4		All Pupils(P)	All Students(S)	Tutorial Staff
S	P	S	P	S	P	S	P			
62	8	21	30	29	13	14	14	17	30	35

'Care of the bereaved' ranks seventh in both stress questionnaires, yet only 41 per cent of both students and pupils had formal instruction in such an area. It is interesting to note that 71 per cent of tutors believed the subject was adequately dealt with. Anticipation of bereavement was clearly not adequately considered, but learners were in disagreement with their tutors, in that 30 and 59 per cent respectively, answered 'yes' to the question of care of the bereaved-to-be in the curriculum. A marked difference between schools again appeared.

A proportion of pupils and students were pleased with their tutors' efforts to prepare them to deal with dying patients and bereaved relatives, the range being between 34 and 6 per cent. Whilst more (20-42 per cent) were 'somewhat pleased', a substantial percentage were 'displeased' (24-73 per cent). Again, tutorial staff were only moderately satisfied with their own efforts in this field and 9 per cent were displeased with their performance.

It would appear that while care of dying patients was not particularly stressed in the curriculum, care of bereaved relatives received even less treatment. It is not surprising, therefore, that an overwhelming majority of learners felt a change in the curriculum should be planned in these aspects of care. Tutorial staff, while not answering so convincingly, did agree that change was necessary (Table 2.6).

Table 2.6: Percentage answering 'yes' to the question: 'Do you consider that teachers should plan curriculum change with regard to (a) care of the dying patient, and (b) care of bereaved relatives?'

	Pupils	Students	Tutorial Staff
(a)	65	71	45
(b)	78	90	59

Traditionally, the responsibilities of doctors and nurses differ in terms of who should tell the patient he is dying. The nurse cannot do so because of constraints placed upon her, and frequently the doctor will not do so because of his lack of preparation in this field. Therefore considerable blurring of responsibility boundaries exist in the multi-disciplinary team caring for the dying patient. There seems to be an unwillingness to draw up written policy concerning the dying patient and his care. In no hospital in the survey was any written policy discovered, and the overwhelming majority of pupils (70 per cent), students (78 per cent) and tutorial staff (90 per cent) stated that there was no policy defining the division of responsibility among physician, nurse, social worker and chaplain, in terms of the dying patient.

Pupils (5 per cent) and students (14 per cent) stated they were often required to write answers to questions about specific care of dying patients; 73 per cent of tutorial staff believe they often required this. However, 42, 53 and 23 per cent of pupils, students and tutors respectively, responded that they rarely required such writing. An alarming 53 per cent of pupils and 35 per cent of students stated they were never required to write on the subject. This deficiency was substantiated in terms of reading required on aspects of care of the dying patient: 14 per cent of pupils, 23 per cent of students and 45 per cent of tutors stated that reading was required. In 100 per cent of cases, pupils and students did not have a specific tutor who specialised in this aspect of care.

No more than 50 per cent of students believed they had been prepared to understand and deal with: the patient's emotional response to dying; the role of denial in the dying patient; the process of the patient's grief; the family's anticipatory grief and mourning; and the nurse's emotional reaction to the patient. Tutors' positive responses to the same items were 73, 64, 57, 68, 77 and 95 per cent respectively.

Controversial issues must be debated if a degree of understanding is to be achieved by professional nurses. These include such aspects as euthanasia, definitions of death, ethics of organ transplant and addiction of terminal patients to narcotics, each of these having a considerable behavioural element. Not more than 26 per cent of pupils and 57 per cent of students remembered being involved in such debates. Tutorial staff once again believed that the items had been discussed. The most extreme example was euthanasia; while 21 per cent of pupils and 57 per cent of students said 'yes', response from tutors was 100 per cent.

It is surely good practice to reach a consensus within a multidisciplinary team relating to dying patients' individual needs. It appears, however, that the students and pupils in my sample pursued their caring role in an almost secluded fashion, with little interaction with other disciplines within the service. The chaplain and social worker seem to have the least interaction with both students and pupils. Only 67 per cent of students and 42 per cent of pupils stated they were encouraged to talk with the doctor, and a similar percentage were encouraged to talk with the family. Forty-nine per cent of students and 32 per cent of pupils were encouraged to talk about social, financial and family problems with the patient. A greater percentage of tutorial staff expressed satisfaction in this area but, of course, the ward sister is the only person who can encourage and maintain such interaction in real and continuous terms.

The neglect of instruction relating to the diagnosis of death has already been referred to, and also its relationship to cardiac arrest. However, 74 per cent of pupils and 96 per cent of students stated they were instructed how to identify cardiac arrest; 95 per cent of tutorial staff responded by stating that they included formal instruction in the curriculum. For some reason, identification of cardiac arrest is not related to the diagnosis of death in the minds of both learners and their tutors. Yet, when the real difficulty is contemplated, namely the discretion to be used as to whether or not to resuscitate the patient, the picture is a dismal one: 29 per cent of pupils and 17 per cent of students did not believe they had been sufficiently instructed, but 67 per cent of tutors stated they specifically included this in their teaching. While 76 per cent of tutors stated they discussed the stress experienced by nursing staff with the learners, only 27 per cent of pupils and 17 per cent of students recalled such instructions.

Sexual Counselling

In discussion with learners at very early stages of training it was often said that sexual counselling was almost non-existent in the plan of care, both in the classroom and in practice on the wards. It was felt, therefore, that a measure of such emphasis would be useful in determining necessary curriculum change.

Fourteen categories of patients were listed in the questionnaire; myocardial infarction in the male and female; mastectomy; hysterectomy; the paralysed; colostomy and ileostomy; cardiac failure in male and female; arthritics; termination of pregnancy; the mentally handicapped; malignant disease; patients mutilated by accident; and the management of ageing male and female patients.

Questions were asked which refer to preparation for sexual counselling as opposed to more general behavioural care. It appears from the collective responses of students and pupils, that the person undergoing hysterectomy was less likely to be neglected in terms of sexual counselling than one undergoing mastectomy. All other responses of students and pupils indicated that this is a field which has not yet been formalised in the teaching programme, thus confirming the verbal reports of learners for every school in my sample. Tutorial responses confirmed the validity of this conclusion.

In terms of general psychological care, the pupils were at a disadvantage in every case. In all but two areas, mastectomy and hysterectomy, a greater percentage of tutorial staff than learners felt the subject to have been adequately dealt with. For pupils, patients undergoing hysterectomy and abortion or those within the categories of mental handicap and accidental mutilation, were particularly vulnerable. Within the field of general psychology, students were fairly well prepared but there was still room for a much greater emphasis.

Only 25 per cent of tutors admitted to writing learning objectives for block periods of study, although there was some evidence that these were beginning to appear in nurse training programmes. This is an area requiring urgent consideration, if education is to be seen by learners to be planned and effective.

Psychology

Overwhelming opinion of both the student and pupil body as to whether they considered enough psychology, that is, behavioural aspects of care, was taught in the curriculum leaves me in no doubt at all that my hypothesis concerning this is validated. Two per cent of pupils and 17 per cent of students believed there was enough psychology taught, and a meagre 36 per cent of tutors. In two schools in my sample, there was a convincing 100 per cent for both students and pupils that psychology was inadequately covered.

Forty-five per cent of tutors believed they were equipped to teach psychology. They were supported in this view by students (29 per cent) and pupils (32 per cent). It is little wonder, therefore, that there were so many evidences of poor preparation. Course content for the preparation of tutorial staff may be the root cause of this problem. The importance of this aspect is discussed in more detail in Chapter 7.

Turning for a moment to the teaching responsibilities of ward sisters rather than tutors; pupils, students and tutors believed the ward sisters to be deficient in the teaching of psychological care – pupils 29 per cent, students 31 per cent and tutors 27 per cent. Teaching method was also a vulnerable area, although the tutors predictably were less confident than the learners that ward sisters were able in this field. Opinion would indicate a high degree of confidence that sister/charge nurse were equipped to teach nursing skills and medical knowledge. The chapters in Section 2 pursue in more detail this issue of the ward sister as teacher.

Anxiety resulting from change of wards is at the eighth position at six months, reducing to 13th position at eighteen months. It was hoped to discover whether senior staff in the hospital appeared to attempt to reduce the apparent stress occurring on each change of ward. Two per cent of students and one per cent of pupils stated that some attempt was made and tutorial staff agreed with their impression. An alarming 29 per cent of students, 35 per cent of pupils and 25 per cent of tutors responded by stating that senior staff never attempt to reduce the stress so occasioned. It is probable that ward sisters had forgotten their own experiences in this aspect. Tutors, however, and in particular those who work in the wards as clinical teachers, must surely take a major part of the responsibility for this deficiency.

The greatest single stress area at eight months is apparently caused when nursing patients in great pain. The nature of pain was, in the eyes of the learners, not dealt with adequately: 22 per cent of pupils and 24 per cent of students believed this to be so. But 90 per cent of tutorial staff considered that discussions were held relating to pain.

Reference has already been made to the practice of disciplining learners in public. This practice ranked second in the order of stress provocation in the stress questionnaire: 20 per cent of tutors, five per cent of pupils and 11 per cent of students stated that no policy existed to prevent such an occurrence taking place.

There seems to be no protection of patients and learners in relation to carrying out procedure before being taught the appropriate skills: 25 per cent of tutors, 19 per cent of pupils and 28 per cent of students stated there was no policy in the hospitals to limit this practice.

According to 41 per cent of students and pupils and 45 per cent of tutors, instruction was given in the nursing care of patients on cardiac monitors – a high stress area at both eight and 24 months.

Once again, the differing practices in the classroom and wards was an area of major concern: 95 per cent of pupils, 73 per cent of students and 91 per cent of tutorial staff stated there was no mechanism to prevent consequent confusion.

In conclusion, there would seem to be abundant evidence that the factors causing anxiety as shown on stress questionnaires were directly related to the curriculum. In many cases, there was agreement between learners and their tutors concerning specific deficiencies, but in others, tutors were under certain impressions that were not part of the learners' conscious experience.

Block Timetables

Another source of curriculum information lies in the actual timetables prepared for learners in block periods of study. Although one cannot be dogmatic concerning behavioural aspects from lesson titles, I looked for a general impression of behavioural care, and weighed this against theory and practice of biological aspects of the course.

In the UK, there is no regulation or recommendation relating to the number of hours to be devoted to the study of psychological aspects of nursing care. There is little doubt that training schools would, in many cases, prefer to deal with psychological factors when discussing specific approaches to specific conditions; for example, would stress the need for careful counselling in cases of pre and post-operative mastectomy.

When analysing the timetables arranged by the schools represented in my research, three out of the four institutions labelled lessons in psychology in the introductory course. Timetables prepared for the rest of training scarcely mentioned psychology as a specific entity but in a few cases there was mention of, for instance, 'the psychological needs of patients with burns'. In only one training school was psychology listed throughout the training period. Tables 2.7 and 2.8 are an approximate assessment of the number of hours spent, in a total training period, on human biology, nursing, microbiology and psychology.

It will be remembered that 36 per cent of tutorial staff believed that enough psychology was taught in the curriculum and only 45 per cent felt qualified to teach the subject. There is little wonder, therefore, that so few references to psychology are to be found in the timetable for general nurses.

One answer may be in the suggestion that a broad-based framework on the subject has never been a feature of general nurse training and therefore tutors are limited in the extent to which behavioural patient care can be emphasised, except in the most superficial of ways. To illustrate the point, it seems that a study of mental defence mechanisms such as regression, repression, sublimation and denial, is an indispensable base on how to observe patient behaviour. Most of the so-called psychology taught in the schools within my research had no such basic framework. It is noteworthy that in Italy, 30 hours of applied and related psychology follows 30 hours of psychological theory, as a mandatory feature of nurse training.

Table 2.7: The total theoretical input for programme for pupil nurses over two years, in hours

	School 1	School 2	School 3	School 4
Human biology	25	15	18	29
Nursing	78	118	116	65
Microbiology	2	4	3	6
Psychology	4	—	4	—

Table 2.8: The total theoretical input for programme for student nurses over three years, in hours

	School 1	School 2	School 3	School 4
Human biology	65	66	53	69
Nursing	140	220	132	187
Microbiology	7	4	7	6
Psychology	5	10	20	6

Portrayal Study

In order to illustrate the value of certain approaches to methodology, one portrayal study is included in this paper. A further seven are contained in the complete thesis (Birch, 1978).

This case study illustrates the following points:

(1) A sudden dramatic rise in the IPAT Anxiety Scale heralds potential disaster. Three IPAT scores are available as follows: 36 (sten seven) in the Introductory Course; 26 (sten five) at point six months; 60 (sten ten) at point thirteen months.
(2) An administrative blunder in terms of industrial relations can seriously compound employees' anxiety. At exit interview the student

reports as follows:

> Ultimately I could not cope with responsibilities which I had
> thought I had wanted. Night duty was the last straw and I became
> disillusioned. When I was an auxiliary it was okay, but as a student
> I felt the patients were not the most important people in the eyes of
> the staff and ward management took precedence. It is mainly the
> students who are not interested in caring for patients. It seemed that
> if an appendix did not have textbook symptoms, a textbook opera-
> tion and a textbook recovery, you were a hypochondriac. The same
> thing was in geriatrics to an extent. There was no physical cruelty
> but there was mental cruelty. Nurses laughed at the patients and
> talked about them as if they couldn't understand — you cannot be
> sure how much they understand! They made fun of them when they
> were sloppy with their eating. You tend to get dragged down and I
> found myself becoming irritable and bad tempered with the patients
> and then I felt guilty . . . I was a bit of a perfectionist — but what do
> you do when you want to do something correctly, like aseptic tech-
> nique, but the trained nurse helping you says, 'You are not practi-
> sing for your assessment — do it this way'?

At exit interview the student was about to undergo a hysterectomy.
Three miscarriages had been experienced before commencing to train.
An unfortunate administrative misunderstanding occurred at the time
the student was forced to take sick leave for a depressive illness just
prior to withdrawal. Three weeks sick leave had already been taken
earlier in training for influenza, following a week of profuse menstrual
loss. The Senior Nursing Officer on the service side of the hospital
wrote to the candidate indicating that as she had not submitted a medical certificate and because the twenty-one days allowed sickness had
already been taken, the student's resignation was required in writing.
In fact the medical certificate had been sent to the student's appoint-
ing officer, namely the Head of the School of Nursing, which was the
correct procedure.

Profile

Reference has already been made to the sudden rise in anxiety levels
to sten 10 at thirteen months of training. A moderately low score on
the Rotter Incomplete Sentences Blank shows that the person is well
adjusted on this test. The following responses, however, indicate that
although well adjusted the subject experiences conflict in the field of

security*:

> *The best* feeling in the world is to be wanted;
> *I need* to be secure;
> *I am very* insecure in new surroundings with strange people.

Comments

The history clearly demonstrates the value of the IPAT Anxiety Scale when there is a sudden dramatic rise in scoring. The subject comments about the apparent secondary place which patients take in favour of ward administration. It could be inferred that the ignorance concerning behavioural care forces nurses into a position where feelings of false security are elicited. If the ward routine is proceeding smoothly it is assumed that all must be well with the patients residing in that ward. Although the student would probably have withdrawn in any case, the administrative blunder added to a clearly devastating experience. Both the withdrawing nurse and her husband felt that this was a particular insensitive error in industrial relations which added to the burden of a person with recognized serious pathological and psychiatric illness. A further technical error relating to the first three weeks of sick time was also made in that the student simply has to make up any time taken over the three weeks and is in no circumstances expected to withdraw merely on these grounds. The student finally withdrew during a severe depressive illness which required admission to a psychiatric hospital.

Conclusions and Recommendations

The main hypothesis stated: 'The pattern of general nurse education produces anxiety in the student and pupil because of its failure to prepare the student and pupil adequately for his/her role in relation to the patient's psychological needs.'

This hypothesis appears to be fully supported by the research from the psychological test results and the reported dissatisfaction with the curriculum as planned by tutorial staff.

Psychological tests do succeed in not only measuring anxiety and conflict levels but in suggesting explicit problem areas to which counselling could be applied.

The sample of students and pupils in this study emerges as a rela-

---

*(full responses are shown in the Appendix)

tively anxiety-ridden group of learners when compared with both Franklin's surgical patients and the general population. The quotations in the early paragraphs of this paper from Revans, the *Nursing Mirror*, and the Report of the Committee on Nursing are substantiated. The Report of the Committee on Nursing states: 'There must be better caring, not least more concern with psychological as well as physical needs, more interest in the individual patient.' This statement seems to be fully supported by the results of the research.

It is recommended that as a matter of urgency consideration be given nationally to a review of the curriculum in relation to its behavioural content. In order to achieve progress it seems that guidance would be necessary to tutorial staff in general nurse training schools to help equip themselves in knowledge of psychological theory. Educational establishments preparing tutors should review their philosophy to provide precise resources to meet the needs of students.

Meanwhile, the practice of teaching psychological care only in direct relationship to specific medical and surgical conditions should be resisted in Schools of Nursing in favour of establishing a positive identifiable core of psychology in the curriculum and building on that foundation by application. The author concludes that this core of theoretical framework should emphasise, among other aspects, the following: Learning theory; Study of personality; Growth and development, including intelligence; Perceptual processes; Human motivation; Conflict and anxiety, with emphasis on reaction to illness by the patient and family; The nature of pain. There is ample evidence that such an awareness would reduce anxiety in the learner, improve the example of trained staff and enhance patient care.

Nurse education cannot proceed any further without an honest re-appraisal of human sexuality in illness. Sexual aspects of behavioural care should be debated as freely as aspects of physical care if we are not to fail the patient at the point of one of his greatest needs.

Aspects of care of the dying patient and bereaved relatives should be explored with every learner and not left to learning by trial and error as appears to happen in the current system. It is the author's personal conviction that this is best carried out by tutorial staff and service staff who have developed clear expertise in this field.

In order to prevent certain learners from being at an advantage or disadvantage relative to their colleagues, it is important that the various responsibilities of the learners and the curriculum to prepare the learners for these responsibilities should be stated in terms of behavioural objectives capable of being evaluated.

Note

1. A sten is a standardised conversion of the raw scores on the IPAT Scale (see Cattell and Scheier, 1963)

Appendix

Responses on the Rotter Incomplete Sentences Blank (Portrayal Study)

(1) *I like* to listen to music.
(2) *The happiest time* is beiu.g with my husband.
(3) *I want to know* many more things about the world in general.
(4) *Back home* was a happy time.
(5) *I regret* having an upset three years ago.
(6) *At bedtime* I like to have a bath and a cup of cocoa.
(7) *Men* can be very childish.
(8) *The best* feeling in the world is to be wanted.
(9) *What annoys* me is insincerity and hypocrites.
(10) *People* often try to be superior in their manner.
(11) *A mother* is the most wonderful thing in the world.
(12) *I feel* very unsure about many things.
(13) *My greatest fear* is bleeding to death.
(14) *In school* I should have worked harder.
(15) *I can't* do many things I'd like to.
(16) *Sports* don't interest me very much.
(17) *When I was a child* I was always loved.
(18) *My nerves* sometimes are shattered.
(19) *Other people* are difficult to get to know well.
(20) *I suffer*.
(21) *I failed* quite a few exams.
(22) *Reading* is a good way to learn.
(23) *My mind* doesn't always retain important things.
(24) *The future* of everyone can never be certain.
(25) *I need* to be secure.
(26) *Marriage* is wonderful for me.
(27) *I am best when* I am with people I know.
(28) *Sometimes* I can be very shy.
(29) *What pains me* is to see a child mistreated.
(30) *I hate* to hear people fighting and rowing.
(31) *This place* is like a second home.
(32) *I am very* nervous in new surroundings with strange people.
(33) *The only trouble* is I can never make up my mind.
(34) *I wish* I could have children.
(35) *My father* is the best father in the world.
(36) *I secretly* would have liked to become an opera singer.
(37) *I*
(38) *Dancing* is one of my greatest loves.
(39) *My greatest worry* is to lose my husband.
(40) *Most women* have a bitchy streak.

References

Birch, J.A. (1975) *To Nurse or Not to Nurse*, RCN, London
Birch, J.A. Anxiety in Nurse Education, Unpublished PhD Thesis, University of
    Newcastle upon Tyne, 1978
Cattell, R.B, and Scheier, I.G. (1963) *Handbook for the I.P.A.T. Scale
    Questionnaire*, Institute for Personality Testing and Ability Testing, Illinois
    Champaign
Franklin, L.F. (1974) *Patient Anxiety on Admission to Hospital*, RCN, London
Hilgarde, E.F. (1966) Foreword in B.E. Levitt (ed.), *The Psychology of Anxiety*,
    Bobbs-Merrill, Indianapolis, New York
Kelly, E.L. and Fiske, D.W. (1951) *The Prediction of Performance in Clinical
    Psychology*, University of Michigan Press, Ann Arbor, Michigan
Lazarus, R.B. (1966) In B.E. Levitt (ed.), *The Psychology of Anxiety*,
    Bobbs-Merrill, Indianapolis, New York
MacGuire, J.M. (1969) *Threshold to Nursing*, Occasional Papers on Social Admin-
    istration, Number 30, Bell, London
Menzies, I.B.H. (1961) *The Functioning of Social System as a Defence against
    Anxiety*, Tavistock Pamphlet No. 3
Nursing Mirror, Editorial 24 March 1977
Report of the Committee of Nursing (1972), Chairman Professor Asa Briggs,
    HMSO, London
Revans, R.W. (1964) Standards for Morale: Cause and Effect in Hospitals,
    Nuffield Provincial Hospitals Trust, Oxford University Press, London
Rotter, J.B. (1950) *Manual for the Incomplete Sentences Blank*, The Psychologi-
    cal Corporation, New York

3 STUDENT NURSES' PERCEPTIONS OF THEIR SIGNIFICANT OTHERS[1]

Bryn D. Davis

Introduction

For the purposes of this chapter, nurse training is seen as a process, the process of becoming a nurse. It has been shown that the relationships between nurse learners and those responsible for influencing them during their training are of great importance (Barnham, 1965; Olesen and Whittaker, 1968; Ondrack, 1975; Mitchell *et al.*, 1972; Lange, 1972; Lamonde, 1974). These relationships are of particular relevance to the development of the professional self-image, socialisation into the role of nurse and the ability to cope with various nursing-related problems.

The nurse learner in this instance was seen as the student nurse, rather than the pupil nurse. In order to prevent the study from becoming too complicated and to keep it to a reasonable time scale, it was decided to restrict the question to that of becoming a nurse through the system leading to registration, rather than that leading to enrolment.

The student nurse was seen as actively interpreting the social system of which she has to be a part during her training, and also that of which she chooses to take part. The other members of these social systems are also making interpretations, and the social system thus has a structure that depends on the relationships between the perspectives of the various participants.

The aim of the study was to monitor the social perceptions of the student nurses during their training and to demonstrate the process of becoming a nurse. This was undertaken by attempting to answer the following questions:

(1) What are the relationships between the student nurses and significant others — those influencing the process of becoming a nurse?
(2) How do these relationships change over time?
(3) How does the professional self-image of the student nurse develop during training?

In order to deal with these questions it is necessary to specify in more detail what is meant by the terms 'relationships' and 'professional self-image'.

The term 'relationship' means the dependencies and perceptions of the student nurses and the shared perceptions between them and significant others. Those aspects to be considered here involve:

(1) The use of significant others as 'resource people' (people to whom the students feel that they can take their problems). To whom did the students feel that they could take their problems?

(2) The descriptions of these resource people by the students.

The term 'professional self-image' refers to the perception of self as a nurse. In particular it involved:

(a) Comparison of the way self is seen as being able to cope with the problem situations with the way that significant others are seen as resource people.

(b) Comparison of the way in which self is perceived as a person and as a nurse with the way in which significant others are perceived.

The objectives of the study involved monitoring certain perceptions of the students concerning the people to whom they felt they could take their problems, and concerning their view of themselves as people and as nurses. Certain expectations were derived from the related literature on professional and nursing socialisation. Thus it was expected that the students would say that they would take their problems to the nurse tutor or ward sister. These are the people within the nurse training system who are employed, and in the case of teaching staff, trained, to play this role of resource person. The tutors in particular are expected to have an understanding of the students' needs and their ways of coping with them. However, the literature also indicates that peers, and possibly parents, may be significant resources during training (Hutty, 1965; Olesen and Whittaker, 1968). Finally, it was expected that those chosen as people to whom the students felt they could take their problems would be described in words reflecting more the interpersonal, psychological aspects of their relationship, and also in words emphasising communication and interaction.

With reference to the question of the way in which the students see themselves as nurses, it was expected that they would increasingly see themselves as being able to cope with the various problems they encountered (Olesen and Whittaker, 1968). It was also expected that the students' views of themselves as people and as nurses would increasingly become like their perception of the trained nurses with whom they worked. Finally, it was expected that their views of self and of the trained nurses would become more professional, in that they would use more role-related words in describing them (Merton *et al.*, 1957; Becker *et al.*, 1961; Olesen and Whittaker, 1968; Lifshitz, 1974).

Method

The main technique used in this study is derived from the theory of personal constructs (Kelly, 1955), and details of the method and design are to be found in Davis (1983). The Repertory Grid (Repgrid) consisted of a list of potential significant others or resource people, including self as I am, and self as I want to be (Table 3.1). The respondents were asked to compare and contrast these people in threes, so that bipolar constructs, or description phrases were produced. Twelve such comparisons were made on each Repgrid, producing twelve constructs or phrases for each grid. The Situational Resources Grid (Sitsgrid) consisted of the same list of potential significant others as on the Repgrid, and also a list of problems, produced by the groups of students participating in the study (Tables 3.2 and 3.3). The respondents indicated on the Sitsgrid to which of the people each problem would be taken. Two lists of people were used, as shown in Table 3.1; formal, consisting of professional or work-related people; informal, consisting of professional people and also family and friends. Two lists of problems were used, as shown in Tables 3.2 and 3.3. One list was produced by the students at the very beginning of training in the first week of introductory block; the other was produced after nine months of the student's training, at the end of the period of study.

Table 3.1: Lists of role titles used in the formal and informal Regrids and Sitsgrids

Formal	Informal
Self as I am	Self as I am
Student Nurse	Mother
Registrar	Father
Ward Sister	Companion
Allocations Officer	Best Friend
Houseman	Disliked person
Patient	Patient
Staff Nurse	Staff Nurse
Auxiliary Nurse	Ward Sister
Clinical Tutor	Ward Doctor
Tutor	Tutor
Self as I want to be	Self as I want to be

Table 3.2: The lists of problems generated by the general students, showing those of the main group and those of the two comparison groups. List 1 was obtained during the first few days of training. List 2 was obtained after 9 months of training

Main Group — List 1	Main Group — List 2
Death	Exams and assessments
Old people	Hours of work
Unsocial hours	Money
People in pain	Night duty
Acquiring knowledge	Inadequate senior nurses
Difficult patients	Responsibility
Hurting patients	Getting on with other nurses
Battered babies	Lack of ward teaching
Bed pans	Uncooperative patients
Being in charge	Cardiac arrests and emergencies
Discipline	Fatigue
Fatigue	Theoretical study

Table 3.3: The lists of problems generated by the psychiatric students showing those of the main group and those of the two comparison groups. List 1 was obtained during the first few days of training. List 2 was obtained after 9 months of training

Main Group — List 1	Main Group — List 2
Incontinence	Wages
Violent Patients	Training
Giving injections	Studying
Travel to work	Hours of work
Death and dying	Travel to work
Exams and studying	Institutionalised nurses
Hours of work	Language
Language	Relationships with patients
Pay	Domestic duties
Living in	Ward teaching
Position as a student	Boredom

The Repgrids and Sitsgrids were subjected to a Principal Components Analysis (PCA), which indicates which constructs or descriptive phrases were most strongly related to each significant other, and which resource people and which problems were most important. The important constructs thus identified were then classified into relevant categories (Table 3.4).

Student nurses undergoing training for the general, psychiatric and sick children's registers were involved in the study. For the purpose of this chapter, only those findings relating to the general and psychiatric students will be discussed.

Table 3.4: List of categories used in the content analysis of constructs elicited on the Repgrids, or those selected from a structural (PCA) analysis of the grids

Categories	Explanation
Personal/Psychological	attributes (behavioural of psychological) or a general or personal nature
*Role	attributes of a professional nature or relating to the work situation
Communication	involving talking or confiding
Self image	attributes, behaviour of situations expressly involving self
Authority	attributes expressing positions in a hierarchy, or being in charge or control

*in some instances this category was subdivided into professional role and educational role.

A whole intake of seventeen general students were recruited, nine of whom were monitored over the whole nine-month period of the study, and a whole intake of twenty psychiatric students, twelve of whom were monitored over the nine months of the study. These students completed Repgrids and Sitsgrids on entry to the School of Nursing, during the first week of Introductory Block, and then at three-monthly intervals, to coincide with changes in their programme so that, after nine months four of each had been completed. On the last occasion, two Sitsgrids were completed, one with the first list of problems created on entry, and the other with the second list, created on the last occasion. Each of the groups of students created their own lists of problems, although both agreed on the same lists of potential resource people.

Findings

The findings of the study will be presented in three sections:

(1) To whom did the students go with their problems?
(2) What kind of people were the resource people?

(3) How did the students see themselves, and with whom did they identify as nurses?

To Whom Did the Students Go With Their Problems?

The study of the way in which the students coped with their problems indicated the need for planned provision of support and guidance, and also showed the process of adjustment to the realities experienced, particularly as demonstrated by the general student nurses.

The general student nurses anticipated that they would be able to cope with the various problems to a certain extent themselves. However, student nurse, staff nurse and ward sister were the most important resource people. The allocation of problems to resource people, in anticipation, indicated a perception of those people which accorded with their generally accepted roles, regarding the various problem situations. However, when non-professionals were also included as potential resource people, in the Informal Grids, then self became less important, and best friend and mother tended to replace the professionals. This confirms the expectation that there would be continued, long-term influence from family and friends as significant others. By the time of the last assessment of situational resource people, after nine months of training, mother, best friend and companion predominated as resource people in both the first and second problem lists.

With the psychiatric student nurses, we find an expression of their maturity, confidence and independence. Throughout the period of study, the main resource person was self as I am. This was the result from both the formal and informal Sitsgrids. Student and best friend were also important as peer group support. A less important secondary group of professionals included the clinical teacher.

After the first few weeks of introductory preparation a major readjustment occurred with the general student nurses, which reflected that shown in other studies, when the more naive, idealistic 'professional' expectations were replaced by the more realistic, practical, 'bureaucratic' experiences. Termed 'reality shock' it is perhaps best seen in the present study as the major reallocation of problems to resource people, as is shown in Figure 3.1, where the lines following the courses of selected significant others indicates the changes in relative importance of the professionals over the nine-month period.

In this figure the various potential resource people are indicated, with their weightings showing their importance, as seen by the students in the allocation problems. The central horizontal line indicates a neutral status, and the distances above or below the line indicate relative positive or negative importance as a referent other for help with the problems.

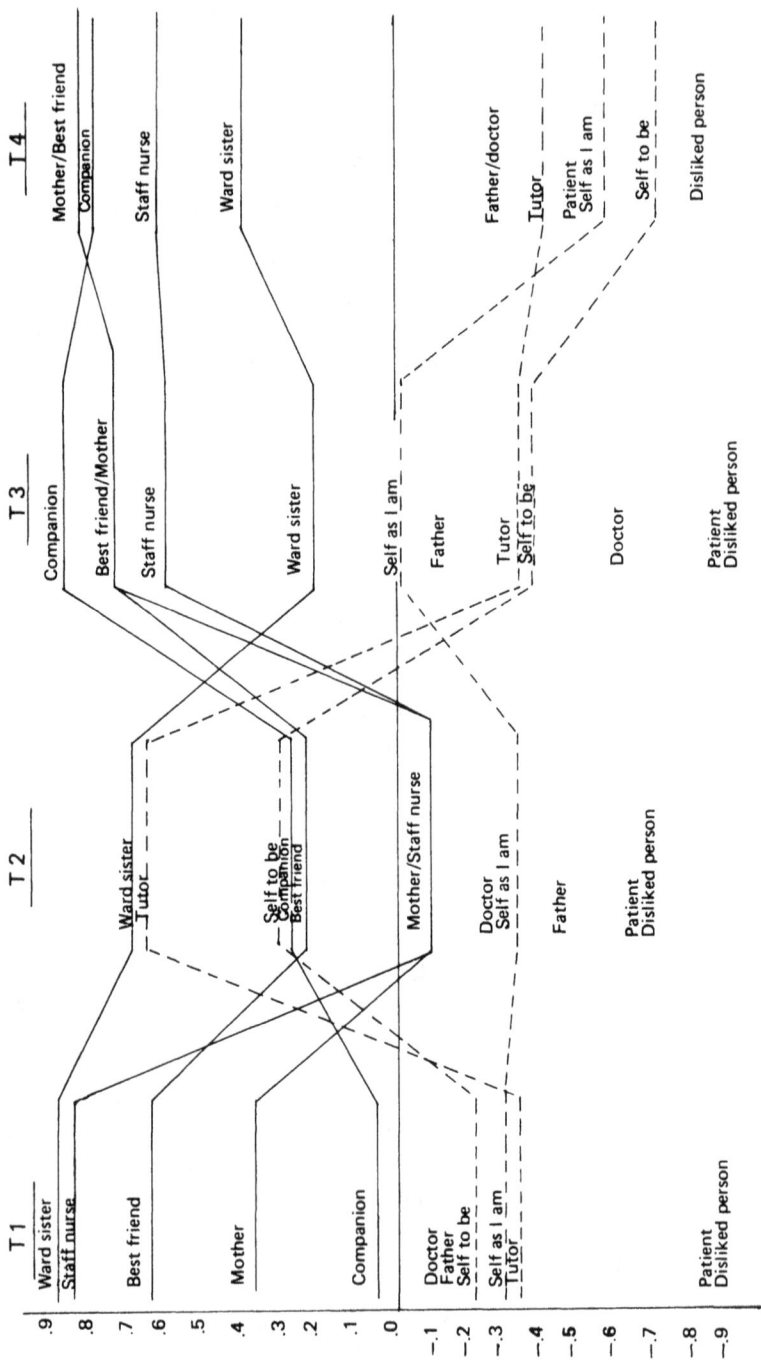

Figure 3.1: The distributions of the resource people along the main component of the general students' informal Sitsgrid on each of the four occasions, showing the relative positions on each occasion.

It must be emphasised that the main point to be made from these findings is that of change and readjustment of resources, and related only to the first component of the PCA (accounting for only a proportion of the total variance – further details of the Principal Component Analysis can be found in Davis, 1983). The actual personnel involved in the changes reflect the feelings of one group of general student nurses. Nevertheless, these findings do confirm expectations derived from the literature.

This readjustment of the general student nurses can be seen as demonstrating their relative naivety and immaturity at the beginning of their course. Many of them had undergone pre-nursing courses, but perhaps they were too young and inexperienced in life to fully utilise their learning from these courses. Alternatively it may have been that these courses were not really relevant to the realities of becoming a student nurse. The predominance of non-professionals over professionals, and in particular over the teaching staff, as resource people, confirms the importance of a well-assessed, planned intervention on the part of the tutors in order to attain and/or retain their role in this respect.

There was no major readjustment on the part of the psychiatric student nurses, regarding the allocation of problems to resource people (Figure 3.2). Compared with the pattern of changes demonstrated by the general students, the psychiatric students made only minor changes, with self as I am predominating throughout the period of study.

This may reflect their maturity and confidence again, in that they were more effectively able to cope with 'reality'. However, most of their problems concerned conditions of work, not ward experiences, and also, living out, they did obtain relief from the hospital-related pressures when they went off duty. The general student nurses tended to spend a lot of off-duty time in the nurses home talking about work and its related problems. It is surprising that their greater tendency to have had previous nursing experience, their frequent discussions with each other about the problems, did not enable them to defuse the 'reality shock' experienced.

Experience may in fact be the key issue. The general students, as mentioned above, were relatively inexperienced both as people and as nurses (young people on pre-nursing courses and cadet training schemes had a relatively sheltered experience of nursing). Knowing about things and talking about them is not the same as experiencing them in general living, as well as in nursing. This is indeed one of the main factors

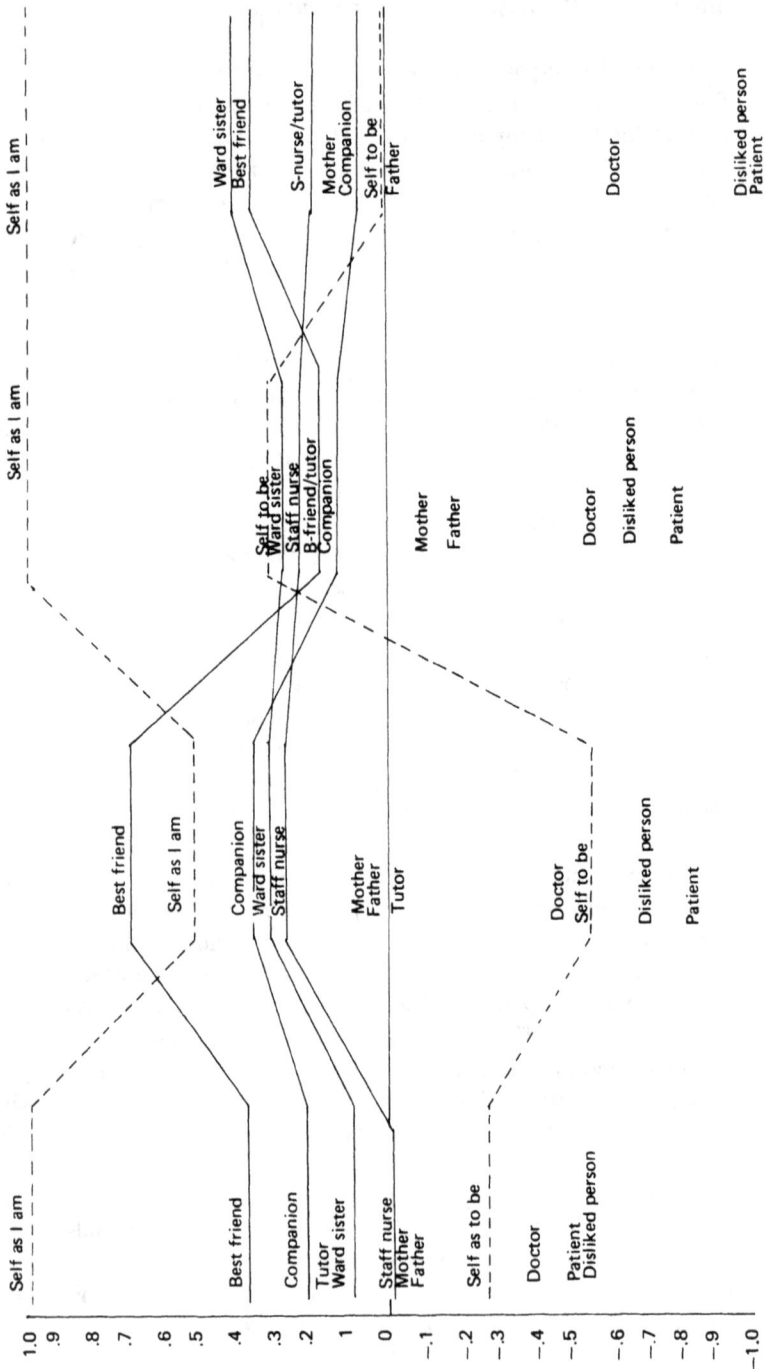

Figure 3.2: Showing the distribution of the resource people along the main component from the PCA analysis of the psychiatric student nurses' informal Sitsgrids and also showing relative changes in distribution over time.

behind the apprenticeship-type of training provided for most nurses. Thus if young people are to be recruited into nursing then adequate preparation and support must be provided. This point emphasises Birch's findings in the previous chapter.

What Sort of Problems Were Taken to the Main Resource People? The major resource people for the general student nurses at the beginning were ward staff, who were seen as being important for problems associated with a general, perhaps naive, view of ward work. The secondary group, teaching staff, were important for problems associated with studying and conditions of service. These of course reflect the students' anticipations, and seem to be related to generalised perceptions of role expectations. When family and friends were included in the range of possible resource people, then they were substituted for the teaching staff in dealing with conditions of service. At the end of the period of study, after nine months, ward staff were seen as important for problems associated with ward work and also acquiring knowledge, examinations and assessments. Mother and friends were seen as important for problems associated with people and conditions of service. Tutor was a secondary resource person, in association with ward staff for problems with examinations and assessments. Thus the ward sister and staff nurse became more important over the nine months of the study, for a range of problems encompassing almost all aspects of the students' world: clinical situations, studying and examinations, and interpersonal problems. Tutor was seen as important throughout for problems concerning knowledge and examinations, as well as conditions of service. Tutor was open to competition, however, from ward staff (sister particularly) regarding acquiring knowledge and examinations, and from mother and friends regarding conditions of service.

With the psychiatric students the major resource people at the beginning of training, self as I am and student, were important for problems associated with conditions of service. The secondary group, ward staff, were seen as being important for clinical problems. This reflects the general role expectations for these people. At the end of the first nine months the same discriminations occurred; however, the clinical teacher became important for problems associated with studying, training and ward teaching. The tutor, in association with the ward sister, was seen as important for interpersonal problems with staff and patients.

This presents a different picture from that of the general students.

On the whole parents and friends were not so important, although best friend maintained a steady level of influence. The other resources were important for problems associated with general role expectations. This difference shows perhaps the different level of maturity of the two groups, as indicated by their ages, time spent in other kinds of work, and the relative importance of self as I am. The mean age for the general students was 19.8 years whereas that for the psychiatric students was 25.2 years. A higher proportion of the psychiatric students had done other work than nursing, whereas a higher proportion of the general students had done pre-nursing or cadet nursing courses.

Changes in the Structure of the Students' Resource System Over Time.
The psychiatric student nurses tended to start with less simplistic, more complex structure than did the general students and the post-registration students. This means that the psychiatric students anticipated a variety of substantial groups of resource people and that the general students anticipated, at the beginning, one major group, and then a variety of much more minor groups. Over time, however, the psychiatric students became more simplistic, having one major group, and then a variety of much more minor ones, whereas the general students moved in the opposite direction. They developed a more complex structure, of a variety of substantial groups of resource people. This was particularly so in the formal setting.

The expectation was that all types of student nurses would become increasingly complex in their systems of resource people and that this would reflect an increased awareness of the nature of the problems and of the help available from various people. There was also the probability of readjustments in relation to increased exposure to the reality of nursing work. These expectations were borne out by the general student nurses but not by the psychiatric students. This presumably reflects their maturity, independence, and more realistic perceptions. Thus even though they did not change their structure in the direction expected, their stability or change was related to their awareness of the nature of the problems and to their accurate perceptions of help available from the various resource people, including self.

What Kind of People Were the Resource People?
The descriptions given by the general students of the professionals chosen as resource people for their problems consist mainly of phrases categorised as Self Image, Professional and Educational Role. The

resource people as shown above were staff nurse, student and ward sister; self as I am, also included in this group, will be discussed below in relation to the development of the professional self concept. It was expected that resource people would be seen in terms relating to interpersonal relations, interaction and communication. However, student nurse was the only resource person seen in terms of Interaction, and that only on the first occasion. Ward sister was seen in Personal/ psychological terms at the end of the period of study, as was the student nurse. In the main, Self Image and Role-related phrases were used by the general student nurses (examples of the words and phrases are discussed below).

When non-professional resource people were included, there was a much greater tendency to describe people in phrases categorised as Personal/psychological, even when describing professionals. Thus at the beginning, ward sister and staff nurse were described mainly in these terms in the informal setting, as was best friend. However, staff nurse was also described in words relating to her Role, both professional and educational. At the end of the period of study, when mother, companion, staff nurse and ward sister were most important, only Personal/psychological words or phrases were used to describe them.

Thus in both formal and informal settings, there was a move from role-related words to those relating to personal attributes. In the beginning, resource people were important because of professional and role-related attributes, as well as for being the kind of people the students wanted to emulate (Self Image), particularly in the formal setting. In the informal setting the resource people were important as people as well as professionals. At the end of the period of study, in both settings there was an increased tendency to see the significant others as being important as people, even though professional attributes were still important for some, for example, the staff nurse. Of course, in the informal setting, the major resource people were non-professionals. The general student nurses seemed to become increasingly dependent on others they regarded as being important as people rather than as professionals.

Within these two major categories, Role and Personal/psychological, the kinds of words and phrases used also demonstrated important aspects of the way in which student nurses perceive their significant others. In the Role category, for example, a frequent point made by the students was that the credibility of resource people was related to their ward experience. Terms such as 'they practise on the ward', 'are on the wards nursing patients', 'will attend to the patient's needs', 'knows the patient closely', indicate that in order to qualify as a significant other, the person must be seen where the action is. Terms such as 'qualified', 'teacher' and 'concerned with nurses' progress', 'instruct nurses who work with them', emphasise the educational characteristics which also help. However, without the ward work attributes, the educational ones are not sufficient (hence the lack of use of the tutor as a resource person). These terms also firmly place the site of the learning process, as seen by the students, as being on the ward, in the practical clinical situation. (See also the Chapters by Ogier, Orton and Gott in Part Two.)

Alexander has recently shown that ward teaching was no less effective than college-based teaching (1982). As it was much preferred by the students in her study, however, and as ward staff felt that ward teaching was more the responsibility of teaching staff, it seems a pity that it does not occur more often. The greater visibility of the teaching staff in the ward setting might also make them more likely to be chosen as significant others by the students.

These recent studies confirm the importance of ward staff, particularly of ward sister as a teaching resource person, as seen by the students, but they also confirm that not much teaching does occur on the wards. As stressed above, the present study was not concerned specifically with teaching, but nevertheless the similarities are noteworthy, and problems of acquiring knowledge were reported as important.

A major difference, however, between these recent studies and the present one is that of the range of potential teachers and resource people. In the present study the importance of ward staff has also been demonstrated, as has the importance of interpersonal relationships in choice of significant others. However, in extending the range of resource people to include non-professionals, there has also been emphasised the vulnerability of both tutorial and ward staff to rejection in favour of, for example, mother, companion and best friend, who were also highly valued in terms of personal attributes, in spite of their lack of professional expertise. This vulnerability was particularly noted with reference to the tutor.

The discussion of perceptions of student nurse resource people has so far included only general student nurses. The psychiatric student nurses in the present study, although seeing self as I am as a more coping person, nevertheless were also dependent on student nurse and best friend. There two roles were described mainly in terms categorised as Role and Personal/psychological. In this case the descriptions of student and best friend involved words and phrases which related to their being also in the process of becoming, but also as being 'involved in ward work', 'caring for patients'. This indicates that best friend was also a professional. As with the general students, the ratio of Personal/ psychological words and phrases increased over time, with that of the role-related terms decreasing. This again confirms the importance of personal attributes in the selection of significant others.

At the beginning of training, the psychiatric students anticipated that ward sister and staff nurse would be important as a secondary group of resource people, but although there were changes over the nine months of the study at the end of the period, the secondary resources accounted for so much less of the variance, that the relative importance of self as I am, student and best friend was greatly increased.

Thus with the psychiatric student nurses we have a picture demonstrating greater self reliance, and also a dependence on peer group support, which is described in terms of similarly being a learner, unqualified, working in the ward, mainly caring for patients' health, and as being nice, compatible, friendly, understanding, caring, and a sensible person.

Some recent studies have attempted to look at the work and attributes of nurse teachers. Sims (1976), for example, reported that a major source of dissatisfaction for teachers was the service-education conflict, as well as staff shortages and pressure work. Tutors particularly were very concerned about their own conditions of work, and, as reported by Sims (1976) and House and Sims (1976), express very little concern for the students' problems, or for their relationships with them. However, one Senior Tutor was reported as noting that 'the profession pays lip service to the needs of students, but ignores those needs in practice' (House and Sims, p. 503). A Principal Tutor was quoted as saying 'it is a very worrying time . . . forced to compromise the nurse in training . . . insufficient teaching personnel . . . they (the learners) are coming into nursing with high expectations and we have to sell them short' (p. 504).

Clinical teachers, who are trained to undertake ward-based teaching providing a link between theory and practice, school and ward, complained that all too frequently they were called upon to replace tutors in the school, and consequently found it difficult to find time to teach the students in the wards. They also reported difficulties in negotiating permission from the ward sisters to teach the students (House and Sims, 1976).

Thus it seems that nurse teachers may very well be aware of their relative unimportance to students as resource people. Their frustration at not being fully responsible for the students' education and training, the conflict between that and service demands, seem to be the major dissatisfaction factors, and must be reflected in a less visible role for them as far as the students are concerned.

How Did the Students See Themselves?

Self as seen by the general student nurses was not a strong concept. Self as I am was not seen as self reliant towards the end of the period of study, when the numbers of constructs correlating highly with self were much lower than at the beginning. Words and phrases categorised as Self Image were a relatively large proportion of the total range at the beginning, with Role-related terms predominating in the formal setting, implying an anticipation of self as being a professional albeit in a learning, untrained capacity. In the informal setting, personal attributes, not professional, were most important. This re-affirms the tendency to see only those with whom a well-established relationship exists in interpersonal terms, whereas professionals were seen mainly on professional terms, unless in comparison with non-professional friends and relatives. Although with the important resource people there had been a tendency to use Personal/psychological terms over time, this did not occur with self as I am. Very little change, apart from the general reduction in the number of constructs mentioned above, was demonstrated. As is shown in Figure 3.1 self as I am and self as I want to be were seen as negative resource people at the end of the period of study, indicating great uncertainty as to the ability to cope themselves and as to their professional self concept. This perhaps reflects the effects of the 'reality shock' experienced a few months previously; alternatively it may be a phase in the search for adequate models on which to base the professional self concept. The oscillation between professional and non-professional resource people indicates this search for significant others as a guide for self development.

This uncertainty was a feature of American medical student training, and undergraduate nurse training. In particular Olesen and Whittaker (1968) described emotional cycles during the process of becoming a nurse, and a great deal of self doubt and uncertainty during the first months in particular, which would be expressed as a group state of anxiety or depression. The fall back on to mother as a major significant other demonstrated this sense of self doubt and a reliance on tried and tested resources with whom warm and supportive relationships existed.

With the psychiatric student nurses Interaction and Self Image were substantial, but minor categories of words used to describe self as I am at the beginning of training. Self Image became more important towards the end of the period of study, whereas Interaction was reduced in importance. In the formal setting Role was the major category, but Personal/psychological increased over time, at the expense of Role, reflecting the change that occurred with the other significant resource people. In the informal setting there were no major changes in proportions of these two categories, both increasing slightly. Communication was not used at all to describe self as I am, and Authority terms only very slightly.

The picture with the psychiatric student nurses seems to be one of self seen as a learner, inexperienced, unqualified, but with a strong self image, and positive personal attributes. The main difference between the psychiatric and general students seems to be this strength of the self image and the importance of interaction.

The expectation for both groups was one of increasing self reliance, only shown here in the psychiatric group, a decrease being demonstrated for the general students. There was also an expectation that the professional self concept would become increasingly like those for trained nurses, as resource people and as nurses. This has not been so. Both groups, at the end of the nine-month period of study still saw self as a learner as unqualified, although the psychiatric group had a stronger self image. Finally it was expected that both groups would come to describe their significant others and themselves increasingly in professional terms. However, as has been discussed above, the increase was in terms of personal attributes, expected to be important for the choice of significant others but not to increase at the expense of professional attributes.

As has been mentioned above, this again illustrates the point that the students, particularly the general student nurses, were in the process of becoming students, as an essential preliminary to becoming nurses. Further evidence supporting this conclusion is that from the study of the students' relationships with staff nurse, discussed next.

With Whom Did the Students Identify? This aspect of the process of socialisation was studied from two directions. The first was an assessment of the statistical relationship between the way the students saw themselves as coping with the problems, and the way they saw staff nurse as coping with them. It was expected that over time the students would come to see themselves as coping with the same kind of problems that they would take to staff nurse. There was little change in distance between self as I am and staff nurse, although the change that did occur was in the direction predicted, and statistically significant for one comparison for the general student nurses. It was also shown that self as I want to be was in all comparisons closer to staff nurse than was self as I am. This perhaps reflects that at that stage of training (nine months) the student nurses were not sufficiently far into the socialisation process to feel themselves as nearer to staff nurse. They seemed to be more involved in the process of establishing themselves as student nurses.

The second approach to studying the models with which the students identified, involved studying the similarities between ways of describing various significant others, and in describing self, in order to identify common parameters.

For the general student nurses there was an increase in the use of Personal/psychological attributes as descriptors and in the identification with family and friends. Thus the importance of personal attributes and of these significant others, as shown with reference to the allocation of problems, is confirmed by this evidence of self being described mainly in the same terms. This of course only applies to the informal setting. However, when the significant others are restricted to professional then the importance of personal attributes is confirmed, and in this context we see that by the end of the first nine months, the tutor was valued by the student nurses regarding personal attributes and self image – 'patient', 'confident', 'more friendly', 'I wish to have the knowledge', 'my ambition', 'I wish to be qualified'.

Of the professional role however, staff nurse was the only one competing successfully with mother, companion, and best friend at the end of the period of study, in terms of Professional Role and Self Image. Also in the informal setting, Communication as a class of descriptors achieved a small but important proportion of the total. This was expected to be a major category of ways of viewing significant others, as was Interaction, but neither reached substantial proportions. It may be that the functions of the words in these categories were embodied in terms classified as Personal/psychological, such as 'friendly', 'understanding', and 'sympathetic'.

Mother became important in terms of Self Image towards the end of the first nine months, at the expense of the ward sister. As mentioned above, this may reflect dissatisfaction with the professionals, but it may also be related to the maturing of the young women and an increasing awareness of their lateral-role socialisation perhaps as married women and mothers themselves. This phenomenon was described by Olesen and Whittaker (1968) for undergraduate student nurses in the

USA and is an important aspect of the development of student nurses during this phase of their lives. Self as I want to be was also described in the same terms as mother regarding Communication and Authority, thus strengthening the evidence for the identification with mother at this stage, although best friend was also described in the same terms.

Another interesting aspect of this study of the student nurses models is that of the importance of the auxiliary nurses, in the Formal setting. Self as I want to be was described in the same Personal and Role terms as auxiliary at the end of the period of study, indicating the influence of their ward experience, during which they spend much time in contact with auxiliaries. The auxiliary was, of course, seen as a resource person with particular reference to dealing with difficult patients, bed-pans and fatigue.

Those role models who had been described by the general student nurses in the same terms as self as I want to be were also, generally, those to whom the students indicated that they would take their problems. However, there were some notable exceptions. Tutor was not chosen as a resource person on the last occasion, but was described in the same terms as self as I want to be. Ward sister and doctor were seen as a secondary resource people on the last occasion, but were not described in terms of self as I want to be.

Thus there seems to be no direct association between being chosen as a resource person and being seen as a person with whom to identify self as I want to be. Tutor, not a resource person, nevertheless is seen as having important Personal and Self Image attributes. Ward sister and doctor seen as important resource people were not seen as having attributes with which to identify, although other important resource people, mother, best friend, and companion were also models for identification of self as I want to be.

With a similar analysis of the psychiatric student nurses' descriptions of self as I am, we find that there is also an increase in the use of Personal attributes, and a drop in the use of Interaction terms, in the Formal setting. Other students and auxiliaries were seen as having the same attributes as self at the beginning and at the end of the period of study. The patient was also seen as having much in common with self as I am, particularly at the beginning, in terms of Self Image, along with student and doctor. At the end of the period, doctor was no longer so important, but ward sister was included, being described in the same Personal and Self Image terms as self. However, when the range of potential significant others included parents and friends, as in the informal setting, no professionals were described in the same terms as self as I am. There were increases in the proportions of Role and Personal terms, and a drop in Interaction terms, although, at the end of the period none of these interaction words were used to describe the significant others. There was also an increase in the proportion of words categorised as Self Image, but again none was used to describe significant others on the fourth occasion at the end of the period of study.

It is surprising that even the Role category did not describe a professional resource person, but only non-professionals. However, when the kinds of words and phrases used by the students in that category are studied, they can be seen to relate to being 'unqualified', 'not a professional', which would be expected of such people as parents and friends.

With the psychiatric student nurses, as with the general students these relationships between choosing people as resources and describing them in the same terms as self, reveal interesting discrepancies. Auxiliary nurse was an important person regarding being identified with self, as were the patient and doctor to a lesser extent. However, none of these was chosen as an important resource person. In the same way, mother, father and companion were not chosen as resources but were important with reference to identification with self as I am. Staff nurse and ward sister were important resource people both at the beginning and at the end of the period of study, and in both the Formal and Informal settings, but they were not described in the same terms as self.

This picture of self described in the same words as family and friends, although these were not chosen as important resources (the exception being best friend), again seems to point to a parallel, lateral socialisation. The psychiatric student nurses, more mature than the general students, had identified with parents and friends over a more extensive period, and continued to do so during their training. They were also in more regular contact with them, as they were more likely to live with them. Professionals were used only as resource people during this first phase of training. However, as has been pointed out above, these students were still only entering the professional socialisation process, and it is quite probable that there would be a change in sources of identification, with professionals playing a more important role at later stages.

Implications for the Process of Nurse Education and Training

In general the process of nurse education and training still embodies a passive role for the learner. Programmes are devised and recruits are required to follow the path laid out for them. Their perceptions, needs and problems have not been considered, in the development of the curriculum, as evidence from studies of the system have shown for at least half a century. Research into nurse wastage has shown that major factors behind withdrawal from training have been poor interpersonal relationships between seniors and juniors, lack of consideration as an individual, repressive conditions of service, and work demands seemingly unrelated to learning needs.

The findings of the present day and of other recent studies discussed above, all emphasise the importance of the learners' perceptions of their experiences, and of the nature and quality of their relationships with their significant others during the process of becoming a nurse. They argue a more active role for the learner, and for the acknowledgement of this in the programmes devised for them.

Many studies have pointed to the need for effective diagnostic assessment of learner's needs and problems (Haward, 1961; Reavley and Wilson, 1972) and Birch has dealt with this issue in the previous chapter, stressing the importance of screening assessments, to prevent the recruitment of unsuitable people. It is an obvious extension of this screening to diagnostic assessment, so that the aim is not to exclude the unsuitable (difficult because the 'suitable' status has not been defined or described), but more importantly, the support and guidance of the learner through periods of vulnerability and stress.

The perceptions of student nurses, revealed by the present study and other studies discussed above, indicate that most recruits, admitted to training mainly on the basis of educational attainment, without the advantage of screening techniques, develop ways of coping, involving the support and guidance of peer, parental and professional significant others (Olesen and Whittaker, 1968; Simpson *et al.*, 1979; Melia, 1982). These studies and the present one show that problems can be identified, stressful situations anticipated and supporting relationships encouraged or developed. In this way, and acknowledging the need for some selecting out of those unsuitable for nurse training (if this could be defined or described) the system is made more flexible, adaptable to the needs and problems of the recruits. This would facilitate a less stressful, more satisfactory socialisation proocess. If the black box of the training system were given elastic sides, so that a variety of people with a range of individual characteristics and attributes could be accommodated; if the learners were treated less like billiard balls, responding passively to prods and cues wielded by the educators and managers; then many of the problems, difficulties and misperceptions described in the socialisation literature, could be alleviated, prevented or dealt with effectively.

Note

1. The research discussed in this chapter was conducted while the author was a DHSS Nursing Research Fellow.

References

Alexander, M.F. (1982) 'Integrating theory and practice in nursing 1 and 2,' *Nursing Times, 78*, Occasional papers 17 and 18, 65-8 and 69-71

Barham, V.Z. (1965) 'Identifying effective behaviours of the nursing instructors through critical incidents,' *Nursing Research, 14*, 65-9

Becker, H.S. *et al.* (1961) *Boys in White*, University of Chicago Press, Chicago

Davis, B.D. 'A repertory grid study of formal and informal aspects of student nurse training,' PhD Thesis, London University, 1983

Haward, L.R.C. (1961) 'A reading comprehension test for nurse learning,' *Nursing Research, 10*, 38-42

House, V. and Sims, A. (1976) 'Teachers of nursing in the United Kingdom: a description of their attitudes,' *Journal of Advanced Nursing, 1*(6), 495-505

Hutty, H.E. 'Student nurses: 1st year problems', MSc Thesis, University of Manchester, 1965

Kelly, G.A. (1955) *The Psychology of Personal Constructs*, Vols I & II, Norton, New York

Lamond, N. (1974) *Becoming a Nurse*, Royal College of Nursing, London

Lange, C.M. (1972) A study of the effects on learning of matching the cognitive styles of students and instructors in nursing education, unpublished PhD Thesis, Michigan State University

Lifshitz, M. (1974) 'Quality professionals: does training make a difference? A Personal Construct theory study of the issue,' *British Journal of Social and Clinical Psychology, 13*, 183-9

Melia, K.M. (1982) 'Students' construction of nursing: a contribution to policy making?', Proceedings of International Conference. 'Research – A Base for the Future?', Nursing Research Unit, Department of Nursing Studies, University of Edinburgh, September 1981

Merton, R.K. *et al.* (1957) *The Student Physician: Introductory Studies in the Sociology of Medical Education*, Harvard University Press, Cambridge, Mass.

Mitchell, V.L., Branach, M.C. (1972) 'Student, faculty and business attitudes towards business and society' in H. Overgaard (ed.), *Proceedings of the Association of Canadian Schools of Business Sixteenth Annual Conference*, McGill University, Montreal

Olesen, V.L. and Whittaker, E.W. (1968) *The Silent Dialogue*, Jossey Bass Inc., San Francisco

Ondrack, D.A. (1975) 'Socialisation in professional schools; a comparative study,' *Administrative Science Quarterly, 20*, 97-103

Reavley, W. and Wilson, L.J. (1972) 'Selection or diagnosis,' *Nursing Diagnosis*, 45-6, 16 November

Simpson, I.R. *et al.* (1979) *From Student to Nurse: A Longitudinal Study of Socialisation*, Cambridge University Press, Cambridge

Sims, A. (1976) 'Teachers of nursing in the United Kingdom: some characteristics of teachers and their jobs,' *Journal of Advanced Nursing, 1*(5), 377-89

Part Two:
TEACHING IN THE CLINICAL SETTING

INTRODUCTION

Bryn D. Davis

During their training, nurse learners spend most of their time in clinical practice, usually on wards, but occasionally in special units or in the community. The process of becoming a nurse is very much related to what happens there. Chapter 3 has indicated the importance of clinical practice in helping the learner to cope with problems and with whom to identify. The three chapters in this section describe studies of the ward environment and of the teaching/learning that occurs there.

The major impetus of Chapter 4 continues the theme of Chapter 3 in attempting to describe the characteristics of an ideal sister as viewed by the learners. Ogier was particularly concerned with the nature of verbal interactions between learners and ward sisters, and with the latters' leadership styles. Also pointed out in the chapter is the importance of the ward sister in establishing and maintaining an environment conducive to learning. As with Chapter 3, Ogier confirms the importance of interpersonal relationships.

In Chapter 5, Orton demonstrates the feasibility of measuring ward-learning climate. She has shown that this existed as a reality for the learners. Particular factors involved seemed to be the sister's perception of learner needs and her commitment to teaching, as assessed both by the learners and by the sisters themselves. This picture is also reflected in other recent studies which have concentrated on the ward as a place for teaching nurses, and on the role of the ward sister in this. Alexander (1982), for example, found that by far the most ward teaching was done by ward staff, with the tutor doing very little. The clinical teacher did some as did the ward sister. Alexander found that staff nurses and students did the most teaching on the ward. She also reported that tutors themselves admitted that they rarely or never taught on the wards. A large majority of students claimed, also, that they learned more on the wards, preferring the ward tutorial as a method of teaching/learning. In a study of students' perceptions of the ward learning environment, Fretwell (1980) found that teaching by ward staff was important, but also that good staff relationships and the ward climate were influential in attaining a good learning environment from observation. However, she found that other students were frequently approached for help, although in interviews the students had claimed that staff nurse and ward sister would be first choice — this confirms the importance of peer group support, as shown in Chapter 3, and at the same time, indicates a difference between intention and behaviour.

In another study of ward climate and its importance for nurse training, Marson (1981) reported that ward sister was seen as the most important resource person, the one from whom the students learnt most in their work experience. Factors influencing this choice included the professional competence of the ward sister, and also whether or not she was seen as communicator, caring about patients, approachable and friendly. This view as echoed by the ward sisters themselves, 76 per cent of whom felt that good relationships, atmosphere and team work were important factors in helping trainees to learn.

In the final chapter of this section, Chapter 6, Gott considers the relationship between preparation in the classroom for clinical experience and learning. She argues that it is particularly important for classroom teachers to be valued by learners at the formative stage of their professional development. This also echoes points made in Chapter 3. Teachers must have credibility in the clinical areas, that is, they must be seen and respected, if they are to influence the process of becoming a nurse, and the level of the standards of care operating there. Gott also demonstrates the importance of communication skills in nursing, and for the training of nurses in those skills.

Thus these three chapters confirm the importance of the dynamic nature of teaching/learning in nurse education. The roles of ward sister and tutor are seen as important in the process of becoming a nurse, not least in terms of their respective credibility, approachability, and the quality of the 'climate' they are able to facilitate.

References

Alexander, M.F. (1982) 'Integrating theory and practice in nursing 1 and 2.' *Nursing Times, 78*, Occasional papers 17 and 18, 65-8 and 69-71

Fretwell, J.E. (1980) 'An inquiry into the ward learning environment.' *Nursing Times, 76*, Occasional papers No. 16, 69-75

Marson, S.N. (1981) 'Ward teaching skills: an investigation into the behavioural characteristics of effective ward teachers,' MPhil Thesis, Sheffield City Polytechnic

4 THE WARD SISTER AS A TEACHER RESOURCE PERSON[1]

Margaret E. Ogier

The research described in this chapter was concerned with identifying the characteristics of ward sisters that might be conducive to nurse learning in the wards. The method of research was an attempt to develop the core of a theory, similar to the method of developing a grounded theory described by Glaser and Strauss (1967).

The particular aspects of the study which will be discussed in this chapter are:

(1) Do nurse learners identify 'helpful' sisters in a consistent manner?
(2) What learning opportunities do nurse learners look for in their clinical experiences?
(3) What learning opportunities do ward sisters identify in their wards?
(4) Is there a mismatch between the learning opportunities nurse learners look for and those which sisters identify in their wards?
(5) Indeed do nurse learners regard themselves as learners or workers?
(6) What are the attributes of a particular sister that can be identified and measured as being conducive to nurse learning?

Do Nurse Learners Identify 'Helpful' Sisters in a Consistent Manner?

Probably every trained nurse can look back over her training and recall a sister or sisters who were particularly influential in helping her training progress. Sometimes it is not easy to say exactly why that person was such a help, was it the way she ran the ward, or took notice of the nurses in training, or what?

To the author, as a nurse tutor, nurse learners appeared to be consistently identifying certain sisters by saying 'sister's good', 'you learn something there' and similar phrases. Was it coincidence that certain sisters were mentioned repeatedly and others were never referred to in this context?

One way of assessing the effect of sisters upon nurse learners was to consider the perceptions of the nurse learner about the ward and sister.

A survey conducted in 1974 of 335 nurse learners indicated aspects within the wards which had had an influence, beneficial or otherwise, upon the learners. As a result of the survey, followed by discussions with nurse learners and trained nurses, certain factors within the wards appeared to be important to nurse learners. Such factors were: sister's approachability, and willingness to answer questions, the fair allocation of nursing experiences and the attitudes of the medical staff and the interest of the tutorial staff.

It was decided to develop a questionnaire utilising the information from the survey, that might be used to measure nurse learners' perception of the ward climate. As a result of the evidence obtained from the survey 27 statements were formed, 26 related to aspects within the ward. One statement was a comparison between wards. For each of the 26 statements five alternative responses (always, often, sometimes, occasionally, never) were supplied. For the comparison statement three alternative responses were provided. The instructions on the questionnaire were: 'Please complete the questionnaire by reading each statement and then placing a tick against the word which most often describes how you feel the statement applies in the ward you are allocated to at present.'

It would then be possible to consider the relationship of the sisters' leadership style, as measured by Fleischman's Leadership Opinion Questionnaire completed by the sister, the sisters' verbal interactions and the nurse learners' perception of the ward climate (LPWC).

The procedural details of the development of the learners' perceptions of ward climate (LPWC) and the suitability of the Leadership Opinion Questionnaire are discussed fully in Ogier (1980).

In order to identify the characteristics of a helpful or 'ideal' sister, 40 student nurses at the end of a three-year SRN training were asked to complete the LPWC questionnaire. The student nurses were tested as a group in the classroom. It was explained to them that a study was being conducted into how sisters managed their wards and that their help was needed in completing some questionnaires.

The questionnaire was used to provide a response profile of an ideal and non-ideal sister for each question. The number of times a particular response was ticked was counted. The response choice for ideal and non-ideal sister for each question could be measured.

All questions were treated in the same way. Questions that had polarised responses to the extent that 65 per cent of the responses were always and often for the ideal sister or occasionally and never for the non-ideal sisters, were identified as 'key questions'. The differences between the questions can be seen in Figure 4.1.

Figure 4.1: The mean scores for 3 groups of 3rd year student nurses who completed the learners' perception of ward climate questionnaire (LPWC) for the ideal and non-ideal sister they had worked with during their training.

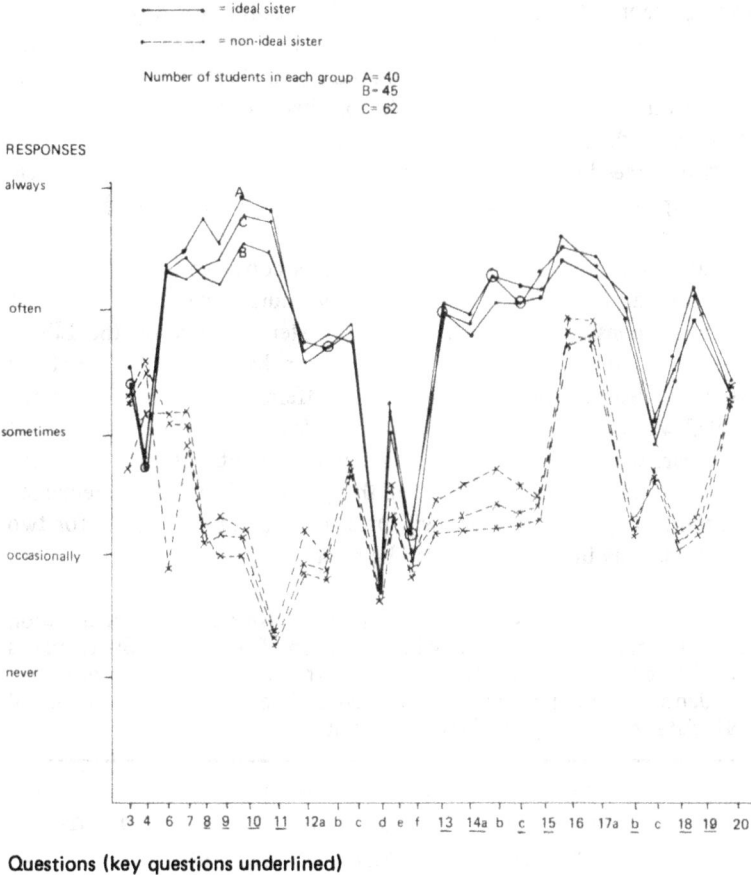

Questions (key questions underlined)

However, as the results had been obtained from one group of third-year nurses who had all followed a closely similar training pattern, had the same tutors and in many other ways had shared common experiences, there was a possibility such a consensus of opinion of an ideal, non-ideal sister profile could be an artifact. Therefore, a year later a further group of 45 third-year student nurses repeated the same procedure. An opportunity arose to make contact with a group of 62 third-year nurses in another unconnected hospital. The student nurses had no knowledge of the research and they completed the LPWC following the same procedure as the first. The results for the three groups are portrayed as a graph in Figure 4.1. In order to portray the results graphically a score is given to each of the five responses: 5 for always, 1 for never. The average scores for each group for each question are depicted in the graph, which also serves to highlight the 11 key questions mentioned earlier. There can be no doubt from third-year student nurses responses to the questionnaire that a profile for their ideal and non-ideal sister developed which was consistent over time and between hospitals.

It becomes impossible to distinguish clearly a graph for one particular group emphasising the similarity of opinions between the groups and hospitals.

Not only did third-year student nurses consistently identify ideal and non-ideal sisters in the same way, nurse learners (pupils and students) consistently rate a particular sister similarly on the LPWC. Over a period of thirteen months some sisters had the LPWC completed by nurse learners in their wards four different times. Each time the LPWC was completed by different nurse learners at different times of the year; when work loads were different, patients different, even the junior doctors were different, yet the profile of each sister remained constant. Table 4.1 and 4.2 will present data for two sisters for two questions only in order to clarify the point.

Table 4.1: The responses of nurse learners in sister B's ward to Question 8, 'Sister makes sure I know what to do' and Question 9, 'Sister makes sure I know how to do what she asks', expressed as a percentage of respondents choosing a particular response. The ideal (I) and non-ideal (NI) sister profile is given for comparison

	February		August		October		I		NI	
	Q8	Q9	Q8	Q9	Q8	Q9	Q8	Q9	Q8	Q9
Always	46.2	61.5	75.0	91.7	25	75	95	85	—	—
Often	38.5	23.1	8.3	8.3	50	25	—	—	—	—
Sometimes	14.4	15.4	16.7	—	25	—	—	—	—	—
Occasionally	—	—	—	—	—	—	—	—	75	72.5
Never	—	—	—	—	—	—	—	—	—	—

Table 4.2: The responses of the nurse learners in sister G's ward to Question 8, 'Sister makes sure I know what to do' and Question 9, 'Sister makes sure I know how to do what she asks', expressed as a percentage of respondents choosing a particular response. The ideal (I) and non-ideal (NI) sister profile is given for comparison

	February		August		October		March		I		NI	
	Q8	Q9	Q8	Q9	Q8	Q9	Q8	Q9	Q8	Q9	Q8	Q9
Always	11.1	22.2	57.1	71.4	40	40	25	50	95	—	—	—
Often	55.6	66.7	28.6	14.3	40	60	25	25			—	—
Sometimes	11.1	11.1	14.3	14.3	20	—	50	25	—	—	—	—
Occasionally	—	—	—	—	—	—	—	—	—	—	75	—
Never	—	—	—	—	—	—	—	—	—	—	—	—

From the data discussed it can be seen that nurse learners did identify helpful or ideal sisters in a consistent manner. Also individual sisters appeared to have been perceived in a remarkably similar way by different nurse learners over the thirteen months they were being studied.

Therefore, it does not appear to be an impression but rather a measurable factor that nurse learners do identify 'helpful' or ideal sisters in a consistent manner. Of the 27 questions forming the LPWC 11 questions were identified as 'key' in differentiating between ideal and non-ideal sisters. The graph in Figure 4.1 shows how the 11 questions polarised the answers. The relevant key questions were:

Q8   Sister makes sure I know what to do.
Q9   Sister makes sure I know how to do what she asks.
Q10   When I don't know something sister makes sure she or someone tells me how to do it or find out about it.
Q11   When I'm worried or don't know something I feel I can go to ask sister.
Q13   Sister makes sure each learner gets a fair share of any learning opportunities.
Q14   If there is a special procedure sister makes sure there is a chance for a learner:
      (a) to watch it
      (c) sister explains it
Q15   I am happy on this ward.
Q17   I feel I can talk to: (b) sister

Q18   Sister is interested in me.
Q19   Sister is helpful to me.

These questions are connected with a sister's approachability and her awareness of the nurse learners and their needs. The two aspects are likely to be interconnected. If a sister appears approachable she is likely to be approached by nurse learners and become aware of their needs, and vice versa.

As nurse learners are so consistent in their views of a helpful or ideal sister, have they got similar expectations of learning opportunities in the wards, indeed do the sisters hold similar opinions about learning opportunities for nurse learners? Perhaps those sisters who are regarded as most or more helpful identify or provide learning opportunities more closely related to the expectations of the nurse learners. These aspects will now be considered.

What Learning Opportunities Do Nurse Learners Look For in Their Clinical Experiences?

To a certain extent a nurse learner's expectations about her next experience will be based upon her present needs, past experiences, future hopes, and a mixture of hearsay and 'formal' information. One of the aims of the study was to try and investigate whether there were any common aspects amongst nurse learners in connection with learning in the wards, and could such common aspects be related to aspects of the ward sisters, management, teaching, supervision or speech. In order to try and sort out any relevant facts three groups of student and three groups of pupil nurses were asked to write down what each nurse learner wished to learn in her next clinical experience. A total of 193 nurse learners generated 740 responses. The responses were sorted using a method of content analysis which resulted in five categories. They are listed below, together with some of the original responses that made up the category.

(1) Theory; includes such phrases as: 'a teaching report; to know *why* something is done not just *how* it is done; discussion with doctors, physiotherapists and the like about a patient's disease and treatment; sister teaches us what she knows; explain a procedure.' Theory category is the 'to know about' category.

(2) Ward; climate includes statements such as: 'I want to work on a

ward where I'm not made to feel foolish if I say I don't know; a ward where I can ask questions; an approachable sister; a ward where I feel part of a team and not just a pair of hands.' Ward climate category refers to the atmosphere of the work environment, friendly or hostile.
(3) Learning accessories; includes reponses such as: 'Textbooks on the wards, management book; charts etc.' Learning accessories includes the tangible and more easily identifiable items that aid learning.
(4) Practical; includes aspects such as: 'to give an injection; to write the Matron's report'. Practical category is the 'to do' category.
(5) Etc. contains responses that are mainly outside the ward environment such as: 'to know what happens in ICU (intensive care unit) so I can understand why the patients are like they are when they get to the ward; to see some of the housing around here.' Etc. category contains items that influence the nurse learner or patient but are not directly related to the ward or fit into the other four categories.

It is assumed that the number of responses that fall into a category indicates the emphasis of response within the category. The results from 6 groups of nurse learners is given in Table 4.3. Besides the number of responses for each group in each category, the percentage of responses in each category is given. The percentage was calculated from the total number of responses for each group considered 100 per cent.
For all nurse learners there is an overall desire for equal amount of theory to practical work.
The difference in emphasis in each category and differences between groups will be discussed shortly. First the perception of the trained nurses in the wards concerning learning opportunities in the wards will be discussed.

What Learning Opportunities Do Ward Sisters Identify in their Wards?

It was possible that the perception of the nurse learners' requirements by trained nurses in the ward was not similar to what nurse learners had expressed as being required.
It was possible to ask two groups of ward sisters, a total of 48 sisters, to list the learning opportunities provided in their wards. They generated 214 responses which were analysed as for the nurse learners' responses and identical categories were generated. However, a difference appears in the emphasis placed in each category, which begins to answer the fourth question of the study.

Table 4.3: The number of percentage of responses attributed to the five learning opportunity categories from 6 groups of nurse learners who responded to the question: What for *you* will be a learning opportunity during your next ward allocation?

	Student Nurses							
Stage of	Beginning		Middle		End		Total	
training	R	%	R	%	R	%	R	% of total for students
Categories								
Theory	61	28	77	41	41	26	179	32
Ward Climate	55	26	15	7	23	15	92	16
Learning Accesses	9	4	16	9	11	7	36	7
Practical	66	31	43	23	60	39	169	30
etc.	25	11	39	20	21	13	85	15
Totals	216	100	189	100	156	100	561	100

	Pupil Nurses								
Stage of Training	R	%	R	%	R	%	R	% of total for pupils	*	†
Categories									
Theory	36	46	6	18	27	40	69	39	248	35
Ward Climate	8	11	9	26	19	28	36	20	128	17
Learning Accesses	0	0	1	3	0	0	1	0.5	37	5
Practical	33	42	18	53	21	32	72	40	241	32
etc.	1	1	0	0	0	0	1	0.5	86	11
Totals	78	100	34	100	67	100	179	100	740	100

*Totals of responses for all learners in each category.
†% of responses in each category from total (740) responses.

R = no. of responses
% = percentage, calculated as described above.

Is There a Mismatch Between the Learning Opportunities Nurse Learners Look For and Those Which Sisters Identify in their Wards?

Sisters generated more responses than nurse learners, the mean number of responses for sisters being 4.5 while the mean number of responses for nurse learners was 3.8.

One reason for the greater number of responses was the specificity of tasks or aspects that the sisters indicated could be learnt in a ward where the nurse learners expressed a more general need. For example, a learner responded: 'to give an enema' where a sister responded: 'soap and water enemas', another responded 'mag. sulph. enemas', yet both sisters' responses were concerned with giving enemas.

In connection with the number of responses in each category, the nurse learners' responses polarise between theory and practical 248 and 241 out of 740 responses respectively, while only half that number of responses was given in the category of ward climate. For sister nearly half (40 per cent) were in the practical category, while ward climate and theory had 26 per cent and 27 per cent of responses.

There is not such a clear polarisation of responses towards theory and practical by the trained nurses as there was for nurse learners. Ward climate is clearly important to the trained nurses. However, the emphasis from the sisters may be seen to be on learning how to do, that is practical aspects of learning.

Of significant interest, especially when the analysis of the sisters' speech is considered, is that the ratio for all nurse learners' responses for theory and practical is a one to one ratio, 248 theory responses and 241 for practical responses. There are slight variations for nurse learners at different stages of training, but the consistent trend of responses is equal number of theory responses to practical responses. The ratio for sisters' responses in the theory and practical categories is 1:2, 43 theory responses to 100 practical responses.

This result might indicate that while in general terms sisters and nurse learners were in agreement about the nature of type of learning opportunities in the ward, the emphasis placed by sisters or nurse learners was different.

One group of ward sisters who have seen these results suggested the reason for the sisters' concern for nurses' learning practical aspects was based on the nurse learner giving service. The sisters' main responsibility was for patient care. The patient care is given largely by nurse learners. Sisters therefore have a concern that nurse learners should know how to perform tasks, as much, if not more, for the patient's wellbeing rather than nurse learners' training requirement.

Nurse learners explained they were concerned to learn how to do the tasks for the patients but frequently expressed the notion that their performance could be improved by understanding the task and its implications. Also theoretical examinations and tests occur at regular intervals during nurse training. These examinations act as a reminder or stimulus to the nurse learners to consider theoretical aspects of nurse training.

The discrepancy between the available learning opportunities, as depicted by the sisters, and the required learning opportunities, as depicted by nurse learners, especially in the category of theory, could indicate an area for potential stress. The categories that have been developed were used to analyse the content of the interview data from ward sisters.

The discrepancy between the ratio of sister and nurse learner responses to theory and practical category might be reflected in the tape-recordings of sister-nurse learner interactions. The following hypothesis was tested during the analysis of the recorded material.

Sisters whose content of interaction with nurse learners is analysed into a ratio of one theory-related to one practical-related interaction will be rated more highly by nurse learners (using the LPWC questionnaire) than sisters whose interaction pattern contains a ratio of theory-related content to practical-related content of one to two or higher.

The testing of the hypothesis and results will be given later.

Do Nurse Learners Regard Themselves As Learners or Workers?

So far I have been using the term nurse learners and sister's influence upon nurse learners, yet in the UK nurses in training do provide a service in the care of the patients. Often the majority of the nurses in a ward will be nurse learners; therefore, is there a role ambiguity, do nurse learners regard themselves as learners or rather as workers? When groups of students and pupil nurses came to the school of nursing they were asked whether on the ward they had just left they had felt like a *learner*; always, often, sometimes, occasionally, never. The question was repeated, did you feel like a *worker*; always, often etc. Altogether five groups of student nurses and three groups of pupil nurses were asked. The results are shown in Tables 4.5 and 4.6.

From Tables 4.5 and 4.6 it can be seen that the majority of nurse learners feel like workers most of the time throughout their training. Interestingly a slightly higher percentage of pupil nurses feel more like learners most of the time; problems arise when a role is unclear or the role expectations of the organisation do not match the role expectations of the individual. Festinger (1957), Aronson and Carlsmith (1962) showed in experimental situations that performance expectancy could affect performance. These ideas have importance for the nurse learner (Kahn *et al.*, 1964), role conflict and role ambiguity is costly by both the person and the organisation, and problems of ambiguity in the work situation are widespread and constitute a source of stress. The main cause for this is the growing complexity of organisations, the rapid technological change and the pervasiveness of certain management practices that foster ambiguity. Nowhere could rapid change fostering ambiguity be said to be occurring more than in a hospital setting. (For further discussion on the role of nurse learners see Ogier, 1982.)

Table 4.5: The percentage of student nurses responding that they always or often felt like a learner L and always or often like a worker W

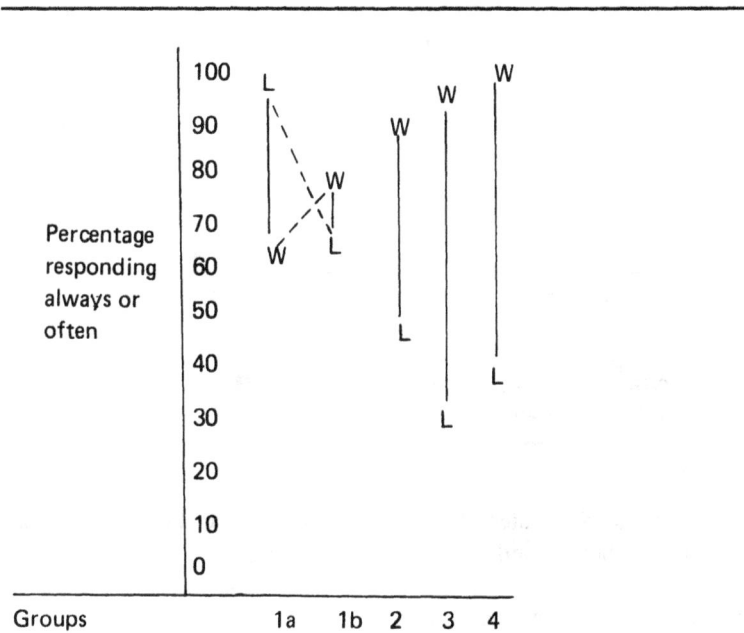

Group: 1a & 1b — 44 student nurses (a) end of introductory course (b) end of first ward
2 — 49 student nurses end of second ward
3 — 51 student nurses end of second year
4 — 40 student nurses end of third year

Table 4.6: The percentage of pupil nurses responding that they always or often felt like a learner L and always or often like a worker W

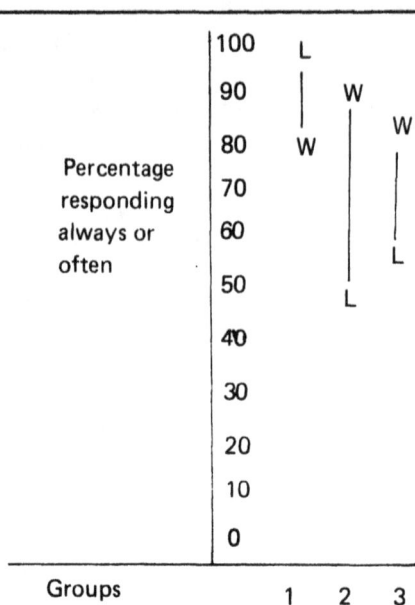

```
             100   L
              90   |    W
                   |         W
              80   W
 Percentage
 responding   70             |
 always or    60             |
 often                       |
                             |   L
              50        L
              40
              30
              20
              10
               0
 Groups            1    2    3
```

Group: 1-17 pupil nurses end of first ward
        2-16 pupil nurses end of third ward
        3-21 pupil nurses end of second year

What are the Attributes of a Ward Sister that Can be identified and Measured as Being Conducive to Nurse Learning?

The most likely time for a sister to have an effect upon a particular learner will be while they are in direct verbal contact with each other. Four ward sisters agreed to be recorded using a radio microphone for a whole week while they were on duty. The way a sister manages her ward and supervises the nurses will also affect the nurse learners, even if less directly. Therefore, the sisters completed the Fleishman Leadership Opinion Questionnaire (1969), which provides two scores that describe the leader's behaviour:

(1) *Consideration*. Reflects the extent to which an individual is likely to have job relationships with his subordinates characterised by mutual

trust, respect for their ideas, consideration of their feelings, and a certain warmth between himself and them. A high score is indicative of a climate of good rapport and two way communication; a low score indicates that the individual is likely to be more impersonal in his relations with group members.

(2) *Structure*. Reflects the extent to which an individual is likely to define and structure his own role and those of his subordinates toward goal attainment. A high score on this dimension characterises individuals who play a very active role in directing group activities through planning, communicating information, scheduling, criticising, trying out new ideas and so forth. A low score characterises individuals who are likely to be relatively inactive in giving direction in these ways.

The verbal interaction of the sisters were analysed in the following ways:

(a) Time spent interacting with various groups of interactors
(b) Detailed analysis of sister-nurse learner interactions:
    (i) direction
    (ii) content
    (iii) form of speech
    (iv) report session analysis
    (v) independent rating by psychologist
    (vi) rating for speech style or manner by psychologists

Nurse learners in the wards of the four sisters completed the LPWC and from the responses it was apparent that two sisters were more highly rated than their colleagues.

For the detailed procedure of the study and results see Ogier (1980, 1982). In this chapter the aspects which distinguish the two pairs of sisters will be discussed.

It must be stressed here that all four sisters volunteered to take part in the study and it could therefore be called a biased sample in favour of nurse learners. The profile for all four sisters resembled that of the ideal sister − two more closely than the other two, hence the rather cumbersome titles 'high-rated' and 'less highly-rated'. It is important to highlight this point for two reasons: first for the sake of the four individuals who so willingly helped − it would be unfair to permit any inference upon their abilities; and second, if differences could be detected in such a favourably biased sample, what differences would have appeared for sisters who expressed views like 'it does not matter what nurse learners think or feel, *I* know what they need to learn in *my* ward and they had better get on with it!'

This study provides significant evidence as to how a ward sister is a teacher resource person. Interestingly the more favoured or highly rated sisters spend less time on duty interacting with anyone! However, when they do interact 40-50 per cent of the interaction is with nurse learners. Toward the beginning of the chapter the learning opportunities in the ward were discussed, nurse learners placing equal emphasis on theory and practical opportunities, while sisters emphasised one theory to two practical opportunities. The categories generated from the learning opportunities were applied to analyse the sister-nurse learner interaction for content. The highly rated sisters had a speech content of theory 14 and 11 per cent, practical 13 and 13 per cent, virtually a 1:1 ratio. However, the less highly rated sisters had a speech content of theory 3 and 5 per cent, practical 11 and 18 per cent, a 1:4 and 1:3 ratio, which follows more closely the opportunities depicted by the sisters for the nurse learners. It could be said that the highly rated sisters were trained staff-orientated in their speech. There is also a noticeable difference in the number of questions the pairs of sisters ask and the number of instructions given. Less highly rated sisters ask twice as many questions but give half the number of instructions. It may be that these two facts are interrelated. Sisters give less instructions so nurse learners are less clear of what or how they should be doing something, necessitating the frequent checking whether tasks are completed. Alternatively both may be a feature of reduced communication, sisters giving less instruction and because of reduced communication channels nurse learners less spontaneously providing or coming forward to sisters, thereby making it necessary for sisters to ask more questions. On analysis of the tapes for one of the highly rated sisters, learners initiated a verbal interaction with sister three times more frequently than for the other three sisters.

From the data collected on the sisters' interaction it might be inferred that the less highly rated sisters communicate less with nurse learners, not only less in quantity but less effectively, in that the content of the interaction is sister-orientated rather than nurse learner-orientated.

The LOQ scores for sisters are clearly related to the preceding data, the highly rated sisters scoring high on Consideration. As mentioned earlier a high score for Consideration on the LOQ is indicative of a climate of good rapport and two-way communication. It is likely that the two-way communications are good and there is a climate of good rapport then the sisters will be aware and sensitive to the nurse learners' needs. This awareness is reflected in the orientation of the speech, in this study highlighted by the 1:1 ratio of theory-to-practical-related speech.

Summary

To conclude, the study discussed in this chapter was an attempt to formulate the core of an emergent theory that would account for the leadership style and verbal interactions of ward sisters with nurse learners. In the context of this chapter it has been possible only to indicate and discuss certain aspects of the ward sister as a teacher resource by facilitating an environment that is conducive to learning. The core of the theory that developed is: ward sisters who have a leadership style that is approachable, nurse-learner-orientated and sufficiently directive for the nature of the work will have a pattern of verbal interaction with nurse learners that is perceived by nurse learners to be propitious to them. It was nearly twenty years ago that Revans (1964) wrote:

> Learning occurs most effectively when doubts in the mind of learners can be voiced spontaneously when they are to him most insistent. If the learner cannot ask questions or seek clarification when he stands in need of it, his learning process will be retarded, since new knowledge is most easily abosrbed when there is eagerness to use it (p. 54).

Hopefully a sister who is approachable and seen to be helpful or ideal will create a climate where nurse learners can progress as Revans indicates.

Lewis (1969) said that research should give rise to practical guides for action. To conclude this chapter consideration will be given to how the information collected in the study described can be used for practical guidelines to enable ward sisters to be active teaching resource persons. There are two main possibilities for action: (a) the provision of structured feedback to assist with behaviour change, and (b) ward sisters' training in leadership and interactive skills.

The Provision of Structured Feedback

Feedback from on-the-job interactions could be utilised by various means; as the study indicated certain aspects of the sisters' leadership style appear to be more appropriate and beneficial than others. Audio or video-recording of the sister could be analysed using a frame of reference from the study. However this is a complex procedure; more simply the LPWC and LOQ could provide sisters with information about their behaviours. At the end of the study the sisters taking part were given feedback on their performances. Several sisters commented how useful and helpful it was to have specific results rather than hearsay or comments from senior nurses. Even a sister who scored low on LPWC showed interest and discussed possible reasons for the nurse learners' perceptions and asked for advice to improve her abilities.

How the Results From the Study Could be Used to Develop a Ward Sisters' Training Scheme With Induction on Issues of Leadership and Interpersonal Skills

The most important aspect is to foster constructive practical interest and concern amongst ward sisters for an improvement in interpersonal skills training, such a need was identified by Lamond (1974).

To conclude, the results of the research described in this chapter can be used in a meaningful way to assist ward sisters to develop an appropriate leadership style with interactive skills that will enable her to fulfil her role as a teacher resource person to the benefit of nurse learners and patients.

Note

1. Much of the research discussed in this Chapter was conducted while the author was a DHSS Nursing Research Fellow

References

Aronson, E. and Carlsmith, J.M. (1962) 'Performance expectancy as a determinant of actual performance,' *Journal of Abnormal Social Psychology, 65*(3), 178-82

Festinger, L. (1957) *A Theory of Cognitive Dissonance*, Raw, Peterson, Evanston, Ill.

Fleishman, E.A. (1969) *Manual for Leadership Opinion Questionnaire 1969 Revision*, Science Research Associates Inc, Chicago

Glaser, B.G. and Strauss, A.L. (1967) *The Discovery of Grounded Theory. Strategies for Qualitative Research*, Weidenfeld and Nicolson, London

Kahn, R.L., Wolfe, D.M., Quinn, R.P., Snoek, J.D. and Rosenthal, R.A. (1964) *Organisational Stress: Studies in Role Conflict and Ambiguity*, Wiley, New York

Lamond, N. (1974) *Becoming a Nurse. The Registered Nurses' View of General Student Nurse Education*, Royal College of Nursing, London

Lewis, B.N. (1969) 'Some troubles with social science,' *Systematics, 17*(2), 139-59

Ogier, M.E. A Study of the Leadership Style and Verbal Interactions of Ward Sisters with Nurse Learners, Unpublished PhD Thesis, University of London, 1980

Ogier, M.E. (1982) *An Ideal Sister? A Study of the Leadership Style and Verbal Interactions of Ward Sisters with Nurse Learners in General Hospitals*, Royal College of Nursing, London

Revans, R.W. (1964) *Standards for Morale: Cause and Effect in Hospitals*, Nuffield Provincial Hospital Trust, Oxford University Press, Oxford

5 WARD LEARNING CLIMATE AND STUDENT RESPONSE

Helen Orton

What went on in sister's ward depended (and still depends) on sister and sister alone (Bendall, 1975, p. 61).

Over the years nurses have held firmly to the belief that learning on the ward is crucially important for learners and that the ward sister is the key person in this area. Individual professional practice has traditionally been underpinned by these beliefs, based on opinion, personal judgement and experience. In recent years, however, the scope of nursing research has widened to include objective studies of ward learning and the related role of ward sister.

The academic base of the studies has included such disparate areas as sociology, psychology, management and education theory and the resulting body of research-based knowledge has led to a situation where nurses are potentially able to supplement and modify their opinions according to factual evidence. However, this shaping process can take place only where information is presented to nurses in a comprehensible manner.

The research about to be described was undertaken in the light of these two considerations, namely that the judgements of nurses merit investigation and that any results must be channelled back into nursing. Particular beliefs chosen for examination concerned the vital importance of the hospital ward as a learning environment and the all-powerful position of sister.

At the commencement of this study in 1975 there was a singular lack of pre-existing research in the field, resulting in a decision to cast a wide net, in the form of an exploratory study, in the hope of catching a worthwhile haul of information.

By means of a questionnaire 325 student nurses and 44 ward sisters responded to a large number of statements and to some open-ended questions. The resulting data gave rise to the proposition that a ward learning climate *does* exist as a reality for student nurses and that it is capable of measurement. Various dimensions of climate were identified by students displaying a high level of consensus in discriminating amongst wards.

90

Before proceeding to describe characteristics of differing ward climates it is proposed to examine the literature, from the two areas of nursing and organisation psychology, which served to guide the research.

Ward Learning Climate: Relevant Nursing Literature

Despite a lack of existing research into nurse education at the commencement of this project, the work of Revans (1964) stands out as an exceptional contribution to the understanding of hospital relationships. In tackling the question of why some hospitals had higher rates of staff turnover than others he concluded that the quality of human relationships reflected in ward atmosphere was crucially involved. Inadequacies in both the quality and quantity of practical guidance on the wards were positively identified. Much later, the Report of the Committee on Nursing (Department of Health and Social Security (Briggs), 1972) contained further valuable information gathered from 3000 trainees. Many of them expressed dissatisfaction with their own training experiences and wanted to see improvements in the quality of ward teaching. Likewise, Birch (1975) in his study of withdrawals from nursing regarded that more than one third of those who left mentioned lack of ward teaching as a contributory factor. A remarkable 98 per cent cited poor staff relationships. Bendall (1975) recorded wide variations in the amount of teaching from one ward to another.

Discrepancies between ward and school practices have been a perennial source of difficulty for learners. Many studies (including Department of Health and Social Security (Briggs), 1972; MacGuire, 1966; Hunt, 1974) have documented daily occurrences of deviation from taught procedures and the difficulties students experienced in attempting to link theory with practice. Bendall (1975) went so far as to assert that no lasting improvement in nursing education could be expected without a resolution of the conflict between 'real' and 'ideal'.

The contradictory nature of the student role, combining as it does both service and training components, presents a continuing problem in nursing. As far back as 1964 the Platt report (Royal College of Nursing, 1964) identified this issue as 'a major obstacle in the path of progress', and again in 1971 the RCN evidence to the Briggs committee asserted that training and service must be separated. Several authors have pointed to the role conflict inherent in this situation (Anderson, 1973; Lelean, 1973) and suggested that students would favour greater emphasis on the learning aspect of their role.

Despite a shortage of research evidence in 1975 there was certainly no lack of nursing opinion. Particularly evident was the firm belief that 'ward atmosphere' does exist (Perry, 1968; Schurr, 1969) and that a favourable atmosphere is beneficial to students and patients alike.

Undoubtedly, the nursing literature offered a rich source of ideas and opinions emanating from a wide range of practitioners with vast, accumulated experience, but it also signalled the need for a more formalised concept of atmosphere, or climate, especially in relation to those features (as yet unidentified) deemed relevant to nurse education.

In contrast to nursing, however, organisational psychology has generated studies of work climate over a period of time stretching back into the 1950s. For this reason it is admirably suited to the process of codifying and investigating opinions found in the nursing literature.

Climate in Organisational Psychology

As early as 1958 Christie and Merton expressed the view that if climates were to be understood, especially their effect on student learning, methods would have to be developed to describe and compare them. Just such a method was proposed by Forehand and Gilmer (1964) with this definition. Organisational climate is: 'the set of characteristics that describe an organisation and that (a) distinguish the organisation from other organisations, (b) are relatively enduring over time, and (c) influence the behavior of people in the organisation' (p. 362).

Even earlier, Pace and Stern (1958) had produced the first of a series of studies of college environments. They combined an environmental measure with a personality appraisal and succeeded in demonstrating that students' perceptions of their environment were not strongly influenced by personality. This finding represented an important milestone in research because it showed that people's personalities do not materially affect their descriptions of climate.

Payne and Pheysey (1971) developed this approach further in seeking to eliminate employee personality from their measure of business organisation climates.

Hospital wards do, of course, differ from both colleges and business enterprises and caution must be exercised in attempts at relating existing studies to the hospital situation. For the student nurse a ward encompasses both learning and work arena and therefore links two functions in a unique manner.

Just as geographical climate is composed of many facets, so the climate of an organisation may be viewed as multidimensional. The research problem resides in the process of identifying and examining the various dimensions. A number of researchers (e.g. Meyer, 1968; Litwin and Stringer, 1968) have suggested particular facets which they proceed to investigate.

Especially useful, in the nursing context, is the analysis of Campbell *et al.* (1970) which incorporated an examination of a large number of climate questionnaires. The authors identified four characteristics relating to the impact of the organisation on the individual and common to them all, namely: (1) individual autonomy; (2) the degree of structure imposed on the position; (3) reward orientation; (4) consideration, warmth and support. This fourth characteristic has a particular relevance for a study of ward climate in the light of nursing opinions concerning the crucial role of ward sister. It also suggests a link between studies of work and those concerned with leadership styles. Although these two areas (climate and leadership) can be viewed as distinct strands within the common thread of organisational research, they both focus on the manner of supervision in a wide range of work situations and the associated attitudes of subordinates.

As long ago as 1939 Lewin, Lippitt and White described three styles of leadership; laissez-faire, directive and participative. These categories have since been utilised by numerous investigators to carry out empirical studies. Not surprisingly they frequently found that people working for participative leaders displayed the most favourable attitudes towards management. Two renowned studies were carried out at Michigan and Ohio Universities in the 1950s. The Michigan study identified two styles of supervision, labelled 'employee-centred' and 'production-centred'. Employee-centred were said to:

> allow their employees to work out the details of when and how work will be handled. They do not feel the need ... to keep a close check on operations (Katz, Maccoby and Morse, 1950, p. 35).

Across a wide range of employment situations the authors noted a consistent tendency for those people working for employee-centred supervisors to be more satisfied with their work than those experiencing a production (or task)-centred style.

The measurement of leadership behaviour provided a focus for the Ohio group's attention. Originally ten facets of such behaviour were isolated and these were later reduced to two dimensions labelled 'consideration' and 'structure'. The authors explained that:

> Consideration includes behaviour indicating mutual trust, respect

and a certain warmth and rapport between the supervisor and his group . . . This dimension appears to emphasise a deeper concern for group members' needs . . . Structure includes behaviour in which the organiser organises and defines group activities . . . Thus, he defines the role he expects each member to assume, assigns tasks, plans ahead . . . This dimension appears to emphasise overt attempts to achieve organisational goals (Fleishman and Harris, 1962, p. 43-4).

These two dimensions were found to be independent of each other; thus a supervisor could score high on one and low on the other, high on both or low on both. Notably, supervisors were found to be significantly influenced by their superiors.

Following the tenor of the Ohio and Michigan studies Blake and Mouton (1964) carried out research which gave rise to training programmes for managers and other leaders. They developed the premise that two independent aspects of leadership co-exist, one being 'concern for people' and the other 'concern for production' (or purpose). They argued that the best leader would score high marks on each count, thus indicating that both consideration and structure are important influences on employee performance and satisfaction.

Large numbers of researchers have devoted their attention to an examination of the environmental context in which the leadership role is exercised (e.g. Payne, Fineman and Wall, 1976). Goal orientations of leaders were studied by Fiedler (1967) who expressly drew attention to situational factors such as 'environmental stress'. He identified two main goal orientations as one reflecting a need to be successful in task performance and the other relating to good interpersonal relationships. Perhaps his main contribution to the guidance of ward climate research is his proposition that a positive, close interpersonal relationship between leader and subordinate is therapeutic in its effect.

'Consideration' appears again in Likert's (1967) organisation studies in which the importance of supportive relationships is again emphasised. Both his own and other people's research led him to the conviction that:

> The leadership . . . must be such as to ensure a maximum probability that in all interactions and in all relationships within the organisation, each member, in the light of his background, values, desires and expectations, will view the experience as supportive and one which builds and maintains his sense of personal worth and importance (p. 103).

In highlighting the crucial nature of the relationship between superior and subordinate, Likert might well have had the hospital ward in mind.

Several studies have suggested that the climate of the total organisation may bear little relationship to immediate job climate. Questions have been posed regarding the size of the collectivity to which individuals relate in their perceptions of 'work climate'. In the realm of nursing the issue centres on whether nurses recognise their work climate in terms of individual ward or total hospital. Schneider and Hall (1973) were in no doubt about the greater appropriateness of focusing on immediate job climate rather than on the wider organisational setting.

Like the early researchers, Payne, Fineman and Wall, (1976) sought to eliminate the personality factor from measures of climate. They emphasised the distinction between organisational climate and job satisfaction in stating that:

> . . . job satisfaction concerns a person's affective response to his job, while organisational climate is derived from a person's description of what the organisation is like. In the case of climate, the respondent is in effect asked to ignore his personal feelings about the organisation and merely describe what goes on (p. 46).

Finally, the place of consensus in climate descriptions is tackled by only a few authors. Forehand and Gilmer (1964) suggested that the definition of a climate dimension required evidence that it was perceived comparably by a majority of those experiencing the climate. Likewise Guion (1973) argued that the accuracy of a perception should be validated against consensus of perceptions. More specific was Payne *et al.*'s statement that:

> Conceptually, it makes sense to look for some consensus among a population if this is to reflect a characteristic of the environment . . . The predictive validity of an organisational climate dimension may be demonstrable under conditions of, say, 55% and 65% consensus . . . (p. 49).

This review of the literature which served to guide the research has attempted to demonstrate the need to supplement and extend nursing knowledge with findings from other disciplines. Organisational psychology was chosen because it already embraced a wealth of research material and could offer tested methods for defining climate.

Findings of the Research

Existence of Ward Climate

Without doubt the most important feature of the author's research was the clear evidence that ward learning climate exists as a reality for student nurses and that it is able to be measured. Analysis of data from the questionnaire revealed two short scales (or clusters of items) one of which focused on the sister's recognition of student nurse needs and the other on the sister's commitment to teaching. These scales are shown in Tables 5.1 and 5.2. In terms of their ability to discriminate amongst a large number of wards and to elicit consensus from respondents the scales were effective. Two entirely different types of ward were identified with striking clarity. At one extreme were located three wards, subsequently labelled 'high student orientation' and at the other extreme three wards labelled 'low student orientation'. These labels were descriptive of the sisters' attitudes towards students allocated to their wards. These six wards provided the focus of analysis because they alone among eighteen wards met the stipulated research criteria of discrimination and consensus.

Table 5.1: Scale 1 — The ward sister's recognition of student nurse needs. Percentage of student nurse responses by type of ward — high student orientation (HSO) and low student orientation (LSO)

Item	HSO Wards Agree* %	(n = 38) Disagree† %	LSO Wards Agree %	(n = 27) Disagree %	x^2 df = 1
(55) All staff on the ward, from the ward sister to the newest recruit, feel part of a ward team	90	11	30	66	24.24 $p < 0.001$
(81) The ward sister attaches importance to the learning needs of student nurses	84	4	30	59	28.53 $p < 0.001$
(89) The ward sister regards the student nurse as a worker rather than as learner	16	82	65	21	21.68 $p < 0.001$
(91) The ward sister is not concerned about what a student nurse is thinking or feeling as long as she is getting on with her work	5	90	63	36	26.12 $p < 0.001$

*Includes both 'agree' and 'strongly agree' responses.
†Includes both 'disagree' and 'strongly disagree' responses.
  Undecided responses are omitted.

Table 5.2: Scale 2 — The ward sister's commitment to teaching. Percentage of student nurse responses by type of ward — high student orientation (HSO) and low student orientation (LSO)

Item	HSO Wards Agree* %	(n = 38) Disagree† %	LSO Wards Agree %	(n = 27) Disagree %	x^2 df = 1
(68) The ward sister devotes a lot of her time to teaching student nurses	79	18	0	100	46.29 $p < 0.001$
(69) The ward sister has a teaching programme for students on this ward	68	26	19	81	22.17 $p < 0.001$
(85) Ward report is used as an occasion for teaching student nurses	90	8	12	85	44.00 $p < 0.001$

*Includes both 'agree' and 'strongly agree' responses.
†Includes both 'disagree' and 'strongly disagree' responses.
 Undecided responses are omitted.

The hallmark of a high student orientation ward was the combination of teamwork, consultation and the sister's awareness of the physical and emotional needs of her subordinates. Students described the situation as not only meeting their own needs but also those of the patients. The sister was seen to have a teaching programme, herself devoting a considerable amount of time to students, and ward report was used in such a way that it constituted a valuable learning session. Role conflict was not widely experienced by students on 'high' wards despite the fact that nurses generally identify such conflict with the learner/worker dichotomy. They identified 'high' sisters as people who regarded them as learners rather than workers and who attached due importance to their learning needs. Additionally, procedures used in these wards differed little from those taught in the school. Patient allocation and individualised care were seen as the norm in 'high' wards and may have been a reflection of the sister's concern for the well-being of all her charges.

In contrast 'low' wards represented the opposite side of the coin. Teamwork, consultation and ward sister awareness of needs were described as absent or deficient. Students saw themselves viewed as 'pairs of hands' and not infrequently had problems in reconciling differences between ward and school procedures. Teaching was given low priority and many potential learning opportunities were wasted.

These ward profiles emerged from analysis of student-only data and therefore could be viewed as partial or one-sided. In order to obtain a balanced picture sisters provided information and opinions concerning the ways in which they ran their wards and their system of priorities. Amongst other differences, 'high' sisters allocated far more time to teaching students than did their 'low' counterparts. And when asked how much time they would, ideally, like to devote to teaching, the discrepancy between the two was even greater. Thus, to a remarkable extent, sisters divided themselves according to the two extreme types of ward and confirmed the behaviour described by students. Any fears that students were insufficiently knowledgeable or discerning about their wards to offer a reliable account were largely dispelled by these results.

Student Response to Climate

After describing ward climate students were asked to respond to items investigating their satisfaction with a particular climate, and the result is shown in Table 5.3. Striking differences emerged between the two extreme groups with 100 per cent agreement by students on 'high' wards that theirs was a good ward for learning. Overwhelmingly they were happy with the experience, including the amount of teaching, and felt theirs was a happy ward for both patients and nurses. A negative picture, on each of these facets, was presented by students on 'low' wards.

Table 5.3: Scale 3 — Student nurse satisfaction with ward experience. Comparison of high student orientation (HSO) and low student orientation (LSO) wards

Item	HSO Wards Agree* %	(n = 38) Disagree† %	LSO Wards Agree %	(n = 27) Disagree %	x^2 df = 1
(97) This was a good ward for student learning	100	0	33	67	35.5 $p < 0.001$
(99) I am happy with the experience I have had on this ward	92	3	55	44	16.36 $p < 0.001$
(107) This was a happy ward for both patients and nurses	87	11	41	41	11.20 $p < 0.001$

*Includes both 'agree' and 'strongly agree' responses.
†Includes both 'disagree' and 'strongly disagree' responses.
 Undecided responses are omitted.

Contrasting responses such as these leave little room for doubt concerning the various levels of satisfaction engendered by ward experience. Given the fact of random allocation (i.e. with no individual selection for particular aspects of behaviour or personality) the evidence strongly supports the assertion that the level of student satisfaction is directly related to ward climate.

Implications of the Findings

Urgent calls for change are constantly made by nurses at all levels within the profession, but unless research findings can be translated into action there is every likelihood that the *status quo* will continue. The value of nursing research lies not so much in the evidence provided (though this may be important) as in the application to professional practice in order to bring about planned change.

As discussed earlier, little research concerning ward climate had been undertaken up to the commencement of the present study, but by the early 1980s the situation had changed dramatically, with the completion of several studies relating to the ward sister role (Fretwell, 1979; Ogier, 1980; Marson, 1981). The validity of these and further studies was enhanced by the fact that they all identified (by diverse methods) the crucial nature of the sister role and associated influences within the ward.

An immediate and obvious implication is that all those involved in the education of learners must be made aware of relevant research. Unless they are offered the opportunity to assess findings and discuss implications they are not equipped to make informed decisions involving change. It can reasonably be argued that sisters have a right (and duty?) to know about the ways in which their attitudes and behaviour affect staff, students and patients in their charge.

Despite the inclusion of 'teaching students' in the job description of sisters there is little doubt that this aspect of their role is assigned small importance at interview and initial appointment. Many times the author was told 'we are not equipped or trained to teach', or 'it is something we do as best we can when we can spare the time'. Such a haphazard approach is conducive neither to good teaching and learning nor to confidence on the part of sisters. The latter require to be trained for all aspects of their role before appointment and on a continuing basis while in post. Sisters have expressed a need for more 'teaching and learning appreciation' courses to help them understand learners' needs and develop appropriate teaching programmes. Just as students need encouragement in their efforts to learn, so do sisters need encouragement and help to improve their teaching performance. There is, too, a sense in which the teacher is also a learner.

It is unusual, apparently, for staff from the school of nursing to be involved in the selection of sisters and yet their expertise in the educational field could be used to advantage in this way. An additional benefit would be increased face-to-face contact between school and service sector, perhaps leading to a greater sense of partnership in developing the next generation of qualified nurses.

Selection to a sister post might be based on potential ability to fulfil all the requirements of this wide-ranging role. Research-based knowledge that some attitudes and behaviour patterns are associated with enhanced student well-being is sufficient reason for the candidates' own attitudes to be explored. Knowledge that teamwork and consultation are positively valued by students (and patients) might influence nursing officers, senior nursing officers and others in the process of selecting for ward sister posts.

The reality of ward life often falls far short of an ideal and many wards are constantly understaffed. This fact must be recognised in any discussion of how sisters carry out their role, for inadequately staffed wards may allow sisters little time for teaching. The amount of ward teaching is, however, known to vary considerably between wards where staffing levels are comparable, and this fact cannot be disregarded. Are we asking the impossible of sisters? Is the scope and range of their duties so wide that teaching will almost inevitably be assigned low priority? A decade has passed since Lelean (1973) called for a review of the sister's role as teacher. She asserted that either the sister's work must be reorganised to give her time to teach learners, or else the teaching function must be removed from her sphere and handed over to others.

Whatever may happen in the future, sisters at the present time are clearly in need of help and support with regard to teaching. Suggestions from sisters in post include the need for more study leave, in-service training, up-dating and courses offering guidance in methods of teaching and learning. Surely it is not by chance that so many sisters express lack of confidence in themselves as teachers and a belief that teaching students is mainly the school's responsibility. Some sisters are aware of the particular learning opportunities available in their wards and set them out as written learning objectives. Wider use of this practice is a desirable aim, with its implicit recognition that different wards offer different learning opportunities. Furthermore, if learners are to be successful in taking advantage of these stated opportunities, the ward sister must manage her team in such a way that all staff contribute fully to ward teaching.

In this latter context it is almost axiomatic that if the sister herself displays enthusiasm for teaching then her staff will do likewise. Conversely, a negative attitude by the sister is likely to be reflected in other qualified members of the nursing team. Acceptance by sisters that good ward teaching is likely to be therapeutic for patients may increase their motivation to face up to their teaching role and demand help in its fulfilment.

Help in the form of specific training programmes necessitates evaluation and feedback to participants. Formal encouragement for sisters to teach must be accompanied by independent assessment so that all those involved in training courses are fully able to appraise them. Both teachers and taught are entitled to detailed feedback in order to monitor and modify their own performances. Nursing officers and tutors, too, need information regarding the effectiveness of teaching and learning for which they are, in some measure, responsible.

Perhaps fewer wards should be designated as training wards, with more liaison between the school and service sector in making such decisions. Some schools believe that ward appraisal is merely a charade resulting in the automatic acceptance of the required number of wards in appropriate specialties. Tutors and clinical teachers frequently mention their lack of information concerning the suitability of wards and their desire for more contact with the service sector. They would value closer relationships with sisters and opportunities to offer them more support. One way in which these hopes might be realised is the acceptance by tutors of a definite clinical involvement as part of their job description. There is good reason to suppose that many Directors of Nurse Education would welcome such a move as a means of narrowing the gap between education and service domains.

No-one denies the need for more clinical teachers and tutors. Numbers in post fall far short of establishment figures with the result that clinical teachers spend far less time in the wards than they, and others, deem appropriate. Many school staff have been heard to speak of their ambition to break down the 'them' and 'us' barriers by spending more time in the wards and by reciprocal visits from ward staff to the school.

Attention focuses naturally on sisters and school staff as authority figures immediately identifiable in the student-learning situation. But what about students themselves? Should they accept greater responsibility for meeting their own learning needs? In recent years the academic quality of successful nursing applicants has been rising. It is likely that these students reflect the general tendency for young people to demand more recognition of their needs and status and to be less willing than their predecessors to display automatic deference to authority. A more questioning approach to their superiors is a predictable, and even laudable development. Thus, students are likely to show an increased awareness of their learning needs and to desire a greater share in meeting them. Manifestations of these changes may well be interpreted by ward sisters as threatening and disrespectful behaviour. Learners who ask numerous questions and offer critical assessment of ward practice are not infrequently viewed with strong disapproval. Sisters need to be better equipped to understand this more challenging approach by students and to accept it as a legitimate form of active learning.

During the early stages of questionnaire preparation the author was invited to many meetings with a variety of nurse administrators ranging in number from one or two to fifteen or twenty. By their willingness to spend time communicating their thoughts, including doubts and fears about the research, these same people offered insights which greatly enhanced the author's understanding of nursing relationships. It became apparent that, at all levels within nursing, people tend to defer to more senior colleagues on the basis of position in the hierarchy. This is not to infer that seniority does not usually merit deference, but that the abilities and talents of those occupying less senior positions may not be given full scope for development.

In the context of hierarchy it is useful to consider the part played by senior nursing officers and nursing officers in the ward sister's definition of her role. Their influence is potentially considerable though it must be emphasised that the present research does not offer direct evidence. Empirical findings from organisational psychology make it abundantly clear that the leader's own superior significantly affects the way he/she treats subordinates and that respect and consideration are reflected downwards.

The author was privileged to attend ward unit meetings in three hospitals and thus to observe patterns of interaction between sisters and nursing officers. On occasions the purpose of the meeting appeared to be nothing more than the passing of factual information (often emanating from an outside source) from nursing officer to sisters. Few questions were asked or invited at these sessions and verbal exchanges between sisters were non-existent or minimal. At the other extreme, nursing officers not only gave information but also encouraged questions and discussion. Exchanges between sisters were frequent and were listened and responded to by all those present. Problems experienced by individual sisters were voiced in a trusting atmosphere with advice and solutions readily forthcoming from peers. Active support and self-help were apparent throughout these meetings with the nursing officer providing leadership and assistance. Of course not all unit meetings fall into one of the two extreme groups: many displayed elements of both types. Little imagination is needed to envisage the influence that may be exerted on individual sisters by nursing officers who are, themselves, subject to yet higher authority.

General Implications

If knowledge equals power it is apparent that greater efforts are needed to share the advantages of research findings more widely amongst nurses. Ward sisters, as managers, require up-to-date knowledge and information on which to base their decisions. Other staff and students, too, must be granted access to this knowledge in order to share responsibility within a ward team.

Consistently in recent years good communication and consultation have been identified as vital for the concept of teamwork to have real meaning. Not just at ward level but throughout the nursing hierarchy patterns of communication require to be fostered and developed. At ward level this might be implemented by, for example, the routine inclusion of students in doctor rounds and the use of ward reports as a learning occasion for the whole nursing team. More contact between every sector and grade of nurse appears to be the wish of most members of the profession. Significant numbers of the author's respondents thought that 'nurses are not very good at communicating with each other' and that there was insufficient co-operation between individuals.

Resolution of the learner/worker dichotomy would constitute a vitally-needed step forward in nurse education. Ample evidence exists that students wish to be seen primarily as learners, and that this view is more likely to prevail in 'high student orientation' wards than in their 'low' counterparts.

One suggestion is that 'ideal' ward climates might be identified and then utilised to educate future sisters who would learn from an 'ideal' sister model. A start has been made in this direction with the setting up of training wards to which sisters are seconded in order to learn the teaching aspects of their role.

Over the years wards have generally been organised on the basis of a work ethos that gives primacy to maintaining routines in order that tasks may be accomplished. Apparently, neither student learning needs nor patient well-being are accorded high priority in such wards, but changes in attitude can be discerned in the trend towards abandoning task allocation in favour of individualised patient care. There is every indication that 'good' learning environments are those in which the needs of patients are met by individualised care. In addition, 'good' learning environments can be identified as those displaying teamwork, good communications and a concern for individual students and their learning needs.

With the virtual explosion of research findings during the last three years there is no longer any room for doubt concerning the vital importance of ward climate and the critical involvement of sisters. No longer is it true to claim, as Stevens did in 1961, that the atmosphere of a ward is poorly understood. Research-based knowledge has illuminated the dark areas and mapped out routes for change. A solitary call for action may easily be ignored but a concerted chorus of research voices demands an active response.

References

Anderson, E. (1973) *The Role of the Nurse*, Royal College of Nursing, London

Bendall, E. (1975) *So You Passed Nurse*, Royal College of Nursing, London

Birch, J. (1975) *To Nurse or Not to Nurse*, Royal College of Nursing, London

Blake, R.R. and Mouton, J.S. (1964) *The Managerial Grid*, Gulf, New York

Campbell, J.P., Dunnette, M.D., Lawler, E.E. and Weick, K.E. (1970) *Managerial Behaviour, Performance and Effectiveness*, McGraw-Hill, New York

Christie, R. and Merton, R.K. (1958) *Procedures for the Sociological Study of the Values Climate of Medical Schools*, Columbia University, Bureau of Applied Social Research, New York

Davies, J. (1971) *An Evaluation of First-line Management Training Courses for Ward Sisters in the Manchester Region*, Centre for Business Research, University of Manchester

Department of Health and Social Security, Scottish Home and Health Department and Welsh Office (1972) *Report of the Committee on Nursing* (Chairman: A. Briggs) HMSO, London

Fiedler, F.E. (1967) *A Theory of Leadership Effectiveness*, McGraw-Hill, New York

Fleishman, E.A. and Harris, E.F. (1962) 'Patterns of leadership behavior related to employee grievances and turnover,' *Personal Psychology, 15*, 43-56

Forehand, G.A. and Gilmer, B.J.H. (1964) 'Environmental variation in studies of organisational behavior,' *Psychological Bulletin, 62*, 361-82

Fretwell, J.F. (1979) Socialisation of Nurses: Teaching and Learning in Hospital Wards, PhD Thesis, University of Warwick

Guion, R.M. (1973) 'A note on organisational climate,' *Organisational Behavior and Human Performance, 9*, 120-5

Hunt, J.M. (1974) *The Teaching and Practice of Surgical Dressings in Three Hospitals*, Royal College of Nursing, London

Katz, D., Maccoby, N. and Morse, N.C. (1950) *Productivity Supervision and Morale in an Office Situation*, University of Michigan, Institute for Social Research

Lelean, S.R. (1973) *Ready for Report Nurse?* Royal College of Nursing, London

Lewin, K., Lippitt, R. and White, R.K. (1939) 'Patterns of aggressive behaviour in experimentally created social climates,' *Journal of Social Psychology, 10*, 271-99

Likert, R. (1967) *The Human Organisation*, McGraw-Hill, New York

Litwin, G., and Stringer, R. (1968) *Motivation and Organizational Climate*, Harvard University Press, Boston

MacGuire, J.M. (1966) *From Student to Nurse: Part II. Training and Qualification*, Oxford Area Nursing Training Committee

Marson, S.N. (1981), Ward Teaching Skills – an investigation into the behavioural characteristics of effective ward teachers, M Phil Thesis (CNAA), Sheffield City Polytechnic

Meyer, H.H. (1968) 'Achievement motivation and industrial climates' in Tagiuri, R. and Litwin, G.H. (eds.), *Organization Climate: Exploration of a Concept*, Harvard University Press, Boston

Ogier, M.E. The Effect of Ward Sister's Management Style Upon Nurse Learners, PhD Thesis, London, Birkbeck College, 1980

Orton, H. (1981) 'Ward learning climate and student nurse response,' occasional paper No. 17, *Nursing Times, 77*, 65-8

Pace, C.R. and Stern, G.C. (1958) 'An approach to the measurement of psychological characteristics of college environments,' *Journal of Educational Psychology, 49*, 269-77

Payne, R.K., Fineman, S. and Wall, T.D. (1976) 'Organisational climate and job satisfaction: a conceptual synthesis,' *Organisational Behavior and Human Performance, 16*, 45-62

Payne, R.L. and Pheysey, D.C. (1971) 'G.G. Stern's organizational climate index: a reconceptualization and application to business organizations,' *Organizational Behavior and Human Performance, 6*, 77-98

Perry, E.L. (1968) *Ward Administration and Teaching. The Work of the Ward Sister*, Baillière Tindall and Cassell, London

Revans, R.W. (1964) *Standards for Morale, Cause and Effect in Hospitals*, Oxford University Press, Oxford

Royal College of Nursing of the United Kingdom (1964) *A Reform of Nursing Education* (Platt Report), Royal College of Nursing, London

Royal College of Nursing of the United Kingdom (1971) *Evidence to the Committee on Nursing*, Royal College of Nursing, London

Schneider, B. and Hall, D.T. (1973) 'Towards specifying the concept of work climate: a study of Roman Catholic diocesan priests,' *Journal of Applied Psychology, 56*, 447-55

Schurr, M.C. (1969) 'A comparative study of leadership in industry and the nursing profession Part I.' *International Nursing Review, 16*, no. 1, 16-30

Stevens, L.F. (1961) 'What makes a ward climate therapeutic?' *American Journal of Nursing, 61*, no. 3, 95-6

6 THE PREPARATION OF THE STUDENT FOR LEARNING IN THE CLINICAL SETTING[1]

Marjorie Gott

Much research has been devoted to the study of the education and training of student nurses, the area of study receiving most attention being the relationship between nursing as taught in the school of nursing and nursing as practised on the ward. That was the starting point for the study reported here. As the study progressed, however, it became apparent that there were other areas of concern for nurse educators. It emerged that some students, in addition to feeling that they were not adequately prepared in practical nursing skills, also felt inadequately prepared to respond to patients' needs; they lacked the interaction skills demanded of a nurse. These two sets of skills, the practical ability to perform nursing duties, and the social ability to interact with and relate to patients seemed to the researcher to be fundamental to the art of nursing, and so these two skills were chosen as worthy of investigation.

The choice of what to investigate shaped the investigation. Recording school teaching and ward practice was necessary to compare and contrast the two. It was more difficult to identify the demands made on nurse learners. Many people, including the learner herself, have expectations which they anticipate should be met. Four principal groups were identified who were believed to exert demands on the learner. These were:

(1) The teacher;
(2) The ward manager (staff nurse/sister);
(3) The patient;
(4) The learner herself.

It was therefore considered necessary to obtain the views of members of these groups with regard to the teaching and practice of nursing. The patient's views were considered especially important, as he is the consumer of the service offered.

Once the facets of the study had been identified, it became clear that the central investigation would be into the effectiveness of (a specific area of) nursing education, and that the central question would be: 'Are nurse teachers preparing junior student nurses for their role as a nurse and, if not, why not?'

Method

A pilot study was carried out in the early months of 1978. In addition to examining the research hypothesis 'training schools do not prepare student nurses adequately for work experience', the pilot study was used to test instruments and methods of data collection that were to be used in the main study.

Data collection for the main study began in the autumn of 1978 and continued throughout 1979. Three quite different institutions were studied: a large teaching hospital served by an area school of nursing, a small hospital in an adjoining region serving a mainly rural population, and a medium-sized urban hospital in the same region as the teaching hospital, but in a different area. The nurse-training school serving the small and medium-sized hospitals were both sub-area schools and were 'on site', unlike the area school which was two miles distance from the hospital. The choice of hospitals was deliberate. It was hoped that examination of three quite different nurse-training institutions would show similarities and differences between hospitals.

Prior to collection of data in a hospital, the researcher met and talked with all of the staff who were to be involved. The first person approached in each instance was the Director of Nurse Education.

The methods used to collect data were as follows:

1. Analysis of Introductory Course Syllabus
An introductory course syllabus was obtained from each of the three nurse-training schools, prior to the course commencing. All teaching sessions during which it was believed the teaching of either practical or social skills could occur were identified. The researcher then obtained permission to observe these sessions. The researcher chose not to declare an interest in social skills, as she believed that the declaration of such an interest could influence both lesson content and teacher behaviour. She said, instead, that she wished to learn how people became nurses.

2. Non-participant Classroom Observation
Prior to sessions commencing, the researcher seated herself amongst

student nurses. With the exception of asking and answering questions, she behaved as did the learners.

3. Non-participant Ward Observation
Selected student nurses were observed while working on their first ward of allocation. The researcher generally did not participate in the delivery of care.

4. Interview
Student, teacher, trained nurse and patient subjects' opinions were obtained by use of a schedule which had been devised for the purpose.

Table 6.1 shows the distribution of the sample interviewed. Most of the subjects were also involved in provision of observation data. All of the teachers interviewed were observed whilst teaching, and all but one of the students were observed whilst working on the ward.

Table 6.1: Interview sample (n = 128)

Occupation Role	Hospital One	Hospital Two	Hospital Three	Total
Sister	5	8	5	18
Staff Nurse	10	2	3	15
Trained Ward Staff	15	10	8	*33*
Tutors	5	4	4	13
Clinical Teachers	5	2	2	9
All Teachers	10	6	6	*22*
Students	17	6	10	*33*
Patients	12	14	14	*40*

The Teaching and Practice of Nursing Practice

In recent research, Birch (1975), Brown (1977), Hunt (1974), Dodd (1974), and Abdel-Al (1975) have examined the relationship between nursing practice as taught in the school of nursing, and nursing practice as carried out on the ward. All of the aforementioned studies reported marked differences between school and ward practice. Later studies (Orton, 1981; Fretwell, 1980) have urged that nursing practice should be taught in clinical areas.

In the present study it was found that nursing practice was almost exclusively taught in the classroom, and that nursing practice on the ward bore little relationship to the practices taught in school.

A complete summary of observations made for each of the three hospitals studied is contained in Tables 6.2, 6.3 and 6.4. Tasks have been ranked according to frequency and major deviations between school and ward practice have been noted.

Table 6.2: Nursing practice: findings, hospital one

Task	Frequency	Deviations From School Teaching	
Taking and recording temperature and pulse rate	73	Thermometer inadequately sterilised No tray Not left two minutes Forgotten	6 6 2 2
Position patient (includes get up and back to bed)	66	Not lifting as taught Patient exposed Left unattended	13 3 3
Take and record blood pressure	51	Patient never told what procedure felt like Taken on right arm Rarely requested second opinion (8 times) Sphygmomanometer incorrectly positioned	51 22 12
Oral medicines	36	Name not checked at bedside Tablet left on locker	16 1
Toilet patient (includes empty drainage bags)	35	Not offer handwashing facilities No apron No cover 7, no cover available Nurse did not wash hand after Unsafe patient left on commode	17 8 3 5 1
Talk to/with patients	31		
Meals	30	Nurse did not wash hands before Kept 'dirty' apron on Gave to patient with 'Fluids Only' sign	8 4 1
Drinks	28	Patient given tepid drink (Nurse did not bother to replenish hot milk supply) Patient given no choice	11 3
Pressure area care	22	Sacral area given hard soapy rub Only one site treated, enquired about Egg white and oxygen used	20 13 2
Make empty bed	19	No toe fold Insufficient linen available	19 1
Chart fluid balance	12 'rounds' + 5 individual	Full urinal ignored	2
Collect trays	16	'Dirty' apron on	1
Bath patient in bed	13	No toe folds Patient not offered toilet facilities Bath blankets unavailable Hair not combed Mouth not cleaned Flannel/towel not changed	13 12 11 7 6 6

Table 2 (continued)

Task	Frequency	Deviations From School Teaching	
		Water not changed	4
		Could not change soiled linen	4
		Talked over patient	4
		Patient exposed	3
Bath patient in bathroom	2	(Patient able to attend to own mouth/hair care)	
Walk patient	11	Patient not spoken to	
Prepare and administer injection	11	Patient not told what drug was for	11
		Nurse did not wash hands before	6
		No cover on needle when expelling fluid	6
		Nurse did not break ampoule safely	5
		Nurse did not check whether entered blood vessel	2
Tasks for patients	11		
Feed patient	8	Stood	1
		Kept 'dirty' apron on	1
Mouth toilet/wash	7	All students observed confused about teaching, asked ward staff	
Occupied bed	5	No toe folds	5
		No linen 'skip'	2
		No linen trolley	2
		Left patient to get linen	2
Request specimen from patient	5		
Neurological observations	4	Not taught, supervised by third year student	3
Assist vomiting patient	4	Not taught	
Wash patient	3		
Dextrostix	3	Not taught, did incorrectly	1
Accompany patient to other department	3	Neither verbal nor non-verbal support	1
Move beds	2	Patient (who was in ward) not told	1
Dressings	2		
Adjust rate intravenous infusion	2	Not practised in school	
Admission	2	No explanation of ward layout, staff, routine	2
Clean incontinent patient	2		

Table 6.3: Nursing practice: findings, hospital two

Task	Frequency	Deviations from School Teaching	
Position patient (includes up and back to bed)	64	Did not lift as taught	10
		Brakes not applied	2
		Inadequate care of intravenous fusion	1
Pressure area care	45	Patient's position not changed	11
		Only one site treated, enquired about	7
		Nurse did not wash hands between patients	7
		Rubbed site with soap/cream	7
Take and record temperature and pulse rate	43	Wore 'dirty' apron	3
		No tray	3
		No bag for soiled equipment	3
Toileting including release drainage	38	Patient not offered handwashing facilities	14
		Nurse did not wear 'dirty' (job) apron	7
		Nurse did not wash hands after	2
		Released bag while patient eating supper	1
Drinks	36	Patient refused, nurse respected wishes	2
Serve meals	24	Patients not given the opportunity to wash before meal	24
Make empty bed	23	Not as taught; no toe pleat, ends/sides turned back	23
		Area/equipment not tidied away	6
Talk to patients	18		
Nasogastric aspiration	14	Nurse did not wash hands before	3
Chart fluid balance	14		
Mouth toilet wash	11	Nurse did not wash hands before	3
		Swab too wet	3
		Used stale solution	1
Oral medicines	11	Patient eating dinner left meal	1
Inhalations	9	Patient did not use correctly	6
		Equipment unsafe	5
Dress patient	10	Hair not combed	1
		Dressed while on commode	1
Walk patient	10		
Occupied bed	9	No toe pleat	9
		No linen 'skip'	3
Feed patient	9	Stood	2
Clean set trolley	9		
Bath patient in bed	8	Nails not checked	8
		Hair not combed	4
		Mouth not cleaned	4
		Urinal not offered	2
		Flannel/towel not changed	2
		Water not changed	1
Bath patient in bathroom	3	Hair not combed	1
		Mouth not cleaned	1

Table 6.3 (continued)

Task	Frequency	Deviations from School Teaching	
Collect trays	8		
Tasks for patients	7		
Prepare and administer injections	6	Nurse did not wash hands before Nurse did not clean site	2 1
Test urine	6		
Take and record blood pressure	3	(not taught)	
Eye care	3	(not taught)	
Assist vomiting patient	3		
Check drug with trained nurse	3		
Dressing	2	No white apron Tore bag over sterile field Dirty dressing over sterile field	1 1 1
Bag linen	2		
Prepare food	1		
Lift with porter	1		
Shave patient (face)	1	(not taught)	
Assist doctor	1	Nurse had not seen procedure before	

Table 6.4: Nursing practice: findings, hospital three

Task	Frequency	Deviations from School Teaching	
Take and record temperature, pulse and respiration	55	Thermometers inadequately sterilised Either respirations, pulse rates, or both, not counted for the recommended time	9
Make empty bed	42	No toe pleat (top sheet turned back) Bed not raised No 'skip' No linen trolley Brake not applied Area not left tidy	42 19 19 19 9 3
Position patient (includes up and back to bed)	37	Nurse did not lift as taught Nurse did not change position of drainage bag Nurse did not put blanket over patient's knees	12 1 1
Meals	35	Nurse did not wash hands before serving Nurse made breakfast for patient	5 1
Take and record blood pressures	33	Nurse did not eliminate radial pulse (usually looked at previous recordings)	33
Toileting (includes empty drainage)	31	Patient not allowed to wash hands Nurse did not wash hands afterwards Full urinals on locker top ignored	27 7 5

Table 6.4 (continued)

Task	Frequency	Deviations from School Teaching	
Pressure area care	27	Sites other than sacral not treated or enquired about	9
		Sites rubbed with soap/cream	15
		Nurse did not wash hands between patients	5
		Nurse did not wash hands after task	5
		Talked over patient	4
		Used egg white and oxygen therapy	4
		Visibly grimy trolley cleaned neither before nor after use	2
Drinks	23	Patients had not been sent what they had requested, nurse made the drinks they had asked for	3
Tasks for patients	19		
Talk to patients	18		
Collect trays	16		
Bath patient in bathroom	12	Mouth not attended to	11
		Hair not combed	6
		No lifting aids, patient too heavy for nurses to lift	3
		Long dirty nails left unattended	2
Bath patient in bed	8	No scissors on trolley/nails not attended to	8
		Mouth not cleaned	5
		Hair not combed	4
		Urinal not offered	4
		Water not changed	4
		Flannel/towel not changed	6
		Nurse did not wash hands after	3
		Nurse did not wash groin	1
		Nurse washed groin of capable embarrassed male	1
Admit patient	8	Two introductory course nurses 'split' duties, one did clerking, the other measurements and recordings	8
		Patient questioned with thermometer in mouth	2
Walk patient	8		
Oral medicines	8		
Care of intravenous infusion	6	Changed bag	2
Mouth toilet/wash	6	Swab too wet	4
Wash patient	6	Nurse did not comb hair	3
		Poor patient made comfortable and left to rest	1
Dress patient	4	Nurse did not comb hair	1
Occupied bed	4	Not as taught	4
		Cradle (not shown in school)	1
Test urines	4		
Dressings	4		
Comb patient's hair	3		

Table 6.4 (Continued)

Task	Frequency	Deviations from School Teaching	
Chart fluid balance	3		
Clean sluice	3		
Feed patient	3		
Prepare teas	3		
Shave ('prep') patient	2	Not taught	
Prepare and administer injection	2	Changed syringe while needle *in situ*	1
Errand to pharmacy	2		
Wash bowls to patients	2		
Identiband	2		
Facial shave	1		
Oxygen therapy	1		
Inhalation	1		
Bandage limb	1		
Remove venflow	1		
Suppositories	1		
Check stores	1		
Summon cardiac arrest team	1		

The most frequent basic nursing duties that student nurses were observed to perform on the wards were bedmaking, pressure area care, toileting and bathing patients.

Bedmaking was never performed as taught. All teachers had instructed learners to insert a toe pleat in the top sheet when making up a bed, but in practice the top sheet was either folded back, or the end of the bed left open. Bedding was also frequently folded under, or back, at one side, as it had been found that this facilitated returning a patient to bed with the minimum of inconvenience (for either patient or nurse). 'Special' beds had been taught by teachers at school three for nursing orthopaedic patients requiring a bed 'cradle'. This style of bedmaking was never seen in practice. One reason for this may be that the type of cradle used in the school was rarely seen on the ward; another reason could be that the 'school way' was lengthy, complicated and out-of-date. In addition to failing to heed nurse teachers' instructions regarding how to make beds, learners also failed to heed their instructions about safety precautions (application of brakes, raising and lowering of beds to prevent back injury).

It would seem with this, as with other nursing tasks witnessed, that, if nurse teachers are too intractable in their teaching students may be unable to identify which behaviours are necessary (for patient and nurse comfort and safety) with dogma.

The importance of hygiene when handling toilet equipment had been emphasised by teaching staff at all three schools of nursing and learners had been instructed to allow patients the opportunity to wash their hands following elimination of excreta. In practice patients were rarely offered the opportunity to do so[2]. Microbiology and theories of 'cross infection' had been taught by staff at all three nurse training schools, and yet these theories did not seem to have been understood and applied to the practice of nursing by students when dealing with patients' toilet needs. Perhaps if teaching had incorporated student involvement in collection and culture of specimens from toilet equipment, hands and skin their behaviour with regard to this practice may have been different.

Wide variations in practice were found in relationship to care of pressure areas. Most variations were recorded at hospital one and hospital three. In the majority of instances that care was witnessed at these hospitals, pressure sites were rubbed. This was in direct contradiction to teaching given, but was in line with current ward practice. In over half of the incidents witnessed at hospital one, and a third of those witnessed at hospital three, only one area, the sacral, was treated. Other sites were neither inspected nor enquired about. Pressure area care is probably the most researched aspect of nursing practice, having received research attention for almost thirty years (Hunt, 1981), and yet research findings are not implemented. It may be that nurses are unaware of research findings, or it may be that they are unconvinced by them.

It would seem that nurse teachers have a role in educating practitioners as well as students in the implications and application of research findings. The nurse teachers observed in this study did not fulfil that role. Nurse teacher advice may in any event be disregarded because (a) they do not practise nursing, and (b) the people who do practise it differently.

Another fundamental nursing duty, the bathing of patients, was also rarely practised as taught. The majority of patients bathed in bed (all hospitals) had neither their hair combed nor their mouths cleaned following a bath, and almost two thirds were not offered toilet facilities prior to the bath commencing. Fewer patients were observed whilst taking baths in the bathroom, but the omissions that had been noted with regard to 'bed baths' were also noted with regard to 'general baths'.

Students' failure to practise whole task behaviour may be due to them having received fragmented instruction in school. Although being told to practise whole task behaviour students were not allowed the opportunity to do so during the introductory course, as tasks were taught on different days and, in one instance, were separated by a week (mouth care and bedbathing). It is not suggested that each task could be adequately taught and mastered in one day, but it is suggested that students be encouraged to show whole task behaviour whilst learning. This they can do by learning the principles of the skills involved (either in school on on the ward) and practising the skills on the ward whilst they are seeking to master them. Bathing a patient in bed would develop and consolidate the skills of bedmaking, bathing, pressure area care, mouth care and communication and would encourage development of the concept of whole rather than fragmented patient care. In addition to being sound teaching this strategy would improve standards of care.

In addition to performing basic nursing duties differently from the way in which they had been taught, nurses also performed technical tasks differently. The measurement of temperature, pulse, respiration and blood pressure rates was rarely performed as taught. This finding is interesting, as learners generally regarded these duties as having a higher status and as being 'more important' than the basic *'caring'* duties. One would therefore assume that they would try to perform them as taught.

Opinions expressed during interview concerning differences between school and ward practice indicated that nurses (students and trained staff) did things differently because the school way was sometimes unnecessary, impractical, or out of date. Replies were usually qualified, however, by the nurse saying that if it was basic care she would do it the 'ward' way, but if it was anything important (injections, dressings), she would try to do it the 'school' way. Reasons nurses gave for choosing the school way tended to fall into two main categories. The first concerned their need to pass General Nursing Council Assessments in order to qualify as State Registered Nurses. The second involved the recognition that the recording of physiological measurements was an essential feature of the successful diagnosis and treatment of patients' illness.

Those students (hospitals one and three) who were frequently responsible for taking and recording blood pressure measurements were extremely concerned that they had been allowed neither the time nor the opportunity to become proficient in the skill during the course. That they often were not proficient caused them great anxiety and distress, especially when this realisation occurred in conjunction with the recognition that measurements went unquestioned and were being accepted as correct:

> Whilst the classroom is artificial, there's some things you've got to practise before you do it on patients, and I don't think we had enough practice. I never set a trolley, I hardly touched a piece of equipment. I only got one chance to practise a blood pressure. Dressings was the worst thing. There was so many things to learn about being dirty you couldn't take it all in. I've learnt it on the ward. If I could actually have practised being the dirty nurse it would have been good. I don't think I really understood the principles; I'm not sure I do now (student, hospital one).

> I don't think we got enough practice on taking blood pressures. I was scared stiff. You think, what if I get it wrong?, but the more you do it the better you get (student, hospital three).

The solution to this dilemma would seem to be either (a) allow the students to develop proficiency, or (b) not to teach this skill during the introductory course.

This latter strategy had been employed by teachers at school two who emphasised basic rather than technical skills in the curriculum. This was resented by some ward sisters, who looked to junior nurses as part of a necessary labour force, there often being no one else to perform the task. Interestingly, however, when questioned sisters thought that students should be concentrating on learning basic skills at this stage in their training.

Unlike nurse teachers, ward sisters have to provide a service to patients, and in order to do so they need a skilled labour force. They may recognise that a junior nurse learner is not the best person for the job, but may often be in the situation of having no one else to use. They may, therefore, have some justification in feeling that, until nurse learners fail to be used as part of a labour force, and until other sources of labour are located, nurse learners need training in the skills commonly demanded in the workplace.

Some nursing practices taught (inhalation of drugs and admission of patients) were rarely observed in practice. Neither task, when observed, was practised as taught – in the former patients' safety being threatened and the latter patients' psychological needs ignored. There may be a case for introducing these tasks later in training when student anxiety is lower, and when proficiency in basic skill has occurred.

Some occupational difference was found between nurses and their view of why ward and school ways of doing things differed. Teachers believed that students did things differently because they did not want to appear 'out of line'. Students and trained nurses also gave this reason, but an equal number of nurses believed the school way of nursing to be impractical, unnecessary, or out of date. That some students could not do things the 'school way' sometimes worried them. They therefore recognised some school practices as better than ward practices. The fact that some nurses (mainly teachers) appreciated that students did not wish to feel 'out of line' when working on the wards indicated their recognition of the existence of two separate and contradictory value systems within the hospital. They recognised the values of school staff as professional and concerned with quality of care (regardless of the quantity demanded), and the values of ward staff as bureaucratic (quantity dictating quality).

This situation has been described as 'reality shock' (Kramer, 1974). No evidence was detected, in this study, to indicate that teachers prepared student nurses to cope with reality shock. Whilst teachers may be powerless to change either the bureaucratic value system of the hospital, or service demands of the learner, were they to convey their knowledge of students' dilemma to them, and also spend time working alongside them at the bedside, the emotional trauma which many students suffer could be reduced. It is also possible that this strategy would enhance, or at least maintain, teacher value for the learner.

It was found, in this study, that whilst tutors were generally regarded negatively by learner and service nurses, clinical teachers were regarded positively. Nurses' views appeared to be associated with amount and type of contact occurring between themselves and clinical teachers/tutors, the relevance of what was taught, and where it was taught. Tutors were poorly regarded because they were rarely seen on wards, they did not take account of work constraints when teaching, and they did not teach on wards; 'They don't teach current ward practice because they don't know what it is' (sister, hospital one).

Clinical teachers were seen frequently, they taught on the ward, and, because they were teaching in the real (rather than artificial) work constraints they were valued by learners and trained nurses alike. The message to nurse teachers is clear; if you want to be valued and influence nursing, and thus patient care, you must teach and practise nursing care on the wards. The message, and the problem, is not new. One wonders how much longer nurse teachers will be allowed to ignore it.

Findings from this and previous researches have indicated that the teaching of some nursing practices may be inadequate or unnecessary. There is, however, a danger that when this is recognised with respect to some aspects of nursing care, the teaching of all aspects of care may be disregarded. Nurse teachers have a valid and important contribution to make towards maintaining and developing standards of nursing care. Standards of excellence are necessary for the development of the profession; nursing will not advance while they are ignored. There would seem to be a need for nurse teachers to decide what constitutes safe and adequate care, and to demonstrate and support their decisions in the workplace.

The Learning and Use of Communication Skills

It has been argued that, because nursing is a social profession, nurses need to possess social (interpersonal) skills. This need has been expressed by learners (Quenzer, 1974; Anderson, 1973; Birch, 1979) but not, until very recently, recognised by nurse educators. Nurse teachers' failure to meet this need could partially account for student nurse disillusionment with nurse training school; by failing to meet this need nurse teachers are not preparing student nurses for their role as a nurse.

That patients are dissatisfied with the type and amount of information they are provided with whilst in hospital has been well documented (McGhee, 1961; Carstairs, 1970; McIntosh, 1977; Annual Report by the Health Service Commissioner, 1978-79; Gregory, 1979). It has been suggested that, in order to be rewarded with information, patients quickly learn (from institutional cues) to take on a 'good patient' role (Cassee, 1975; Danzinger, 1976), but that doing so may not be in their own best interests.

In the absence of training in communication skill, student nurses learn to deal with patients in such a way as to prevent close and intimate relationships developing, as these would be a psychological threat to the nurses. It has been argued that this is why nurses nurse patients by a task rather than a patient assignment system of work allocation (Menzies, 1970; Cassee, 1975; Armitage, 1980). Faulkner (1981) has argued that nurses communicate as they do because they have learnt that communicating with patients is not valued by the system within which they work; getting tasks done on time is.

In spite of this behaviour, nursing is generally recognised and regarded as a caring profession and nurse educators (at least) expect nurses, at the end of training, to be socially skilled; they are expected to recognise and deal with patients' and relatives' emotional needs which (because of the milieu in which nursing takes place) may often be very extreme. Why then have communication skills been neglected in nurse training?

An answer may lie in the way in which nurse teachers are prepared. Until very recently teachers of nursing were not themselves educated in the behavioural sciences and so they may have been unaware of the contribution that these disciplines could make to the practice of nursing. Another answer, also concerned with the teaching of nursing, may lie in the way in which nursing is taught.

It has been documented (Report of the Committee on Nursing, 1972) that nurse teachers prefer traditional methods of teaching and teacher-centred, rather than student-centred, learning. The teaching of interpersonal skills demands more imaginative and innovative teaching methods, and student-centred learning. Nurse teachers may find these methods very threatening as students rather than they themselves will control learning. This issue of control is central to nurse education. It has been argued (Dodd, 1974; Bendall, 1975; Pepper, 1977) that nurse teachers control the learning environment as rigidly as they do because they realise that their legitimacy is tenuous in the eyes of both learner and trained nurses, many of whom believe that the only value nurse teachers have is that of enabling learners to pass examinations.

The Teaching of Communication Skills

Psychology lectures were provided in all three schools of nursing and during these, patients' needs, emotions and behaviour were identified. All sessions were presented as lectures and were teacher-centred. Patients' emotions were also discussed, at each school, during some nursing practice lessons, and students were encouraged to talk to patients and to explain procedures to them. On no occasions, however, were they shown how to do so or allowed to explore or practise communication skills. Communication theories were presented in two nurse-training schools (schools one and three) but, again, these were presented as lectures and no practical application was provided.

It could therefore be argued that nurse teachers paid lip service to the need for nurses to communicate with patients, by not allowing time for the practice and development of this nursing skill as part of the planned introductory course preparation (as they did with other nursing skills). As communication skill development was not provided for students during the course the only way in which nurse learners could learn nurse/patient communication skills was to watch how other nurses communicated with patients (use role models). Also, as in all but one instance, nursing practice was taught in school, they therefore had nurse teacher behaviour as their predominant role model. This was unfortunate, as it did not seem that nurse teachers recognised this as part of their teaching function and rarely addressed communications to a 'patient'.

At school one a doll was used to teach aspects of nursing practice and, in the majority of instances, it was not spoken to, both teachers and learners seeing talking to a doll as 'silly'. On four of the occasions that it was addressed, however, communications were inhibitive to the communication process, being commanding, discouraging and superficial. They were as follows: 'Close your eyes sweetheart'; 'Just lie back and relax dear'; 'All right dear?' (after procedure); 'Pop that under your tongue, lovely'. These communications were associated with negative non-verbal cues (such as walking away).

The other communication was used by a clinical teacher when a small group of students were practising washing/bathing a patient: 'Now nurse – how do you feel?'; 'Do you feel dry?'; 'Are you comfortable?'; 'Do you feel refreshed?'; 'Is there anything that you'd like to say?' This communication was classed as facilitative to the communication process, being open, encouraging and specific to that individual 'patient'.

A doll was not used at school two, as a student role played a patient when one was required. A wider range of communication styles was exhibited here but, again, they were principally inhibitive to the communication process. Unlike students at the other two nurse training schools, students at school two were involved in learning some nursing practice on the wards (the giving of oral medicines). They were, therefore, able to learn how the teacher communicated with the patients she was administering medicines to. With one exception her style was inhibitive (six occasions). It was therefore possible that, because students were witnessing ideal (nursing practice) behaviour they may have believed that the teacher was also demonstrating ideal communication behaviour. As the communication behaviour of students was neither encouraged, explored nor tested by nurse educators, there is no way of knowing whether or not they did, in fact, use this teacher as a role model for communication behaviour.

It would seem that, whatever nurse teachers say to student nurses regarding the value of communicating with patients is unlikely to be regarded by students unless they see the advice put into practice. This was forceably demonstrated by students at school three who, when asked by a teacher what was the first thing they should do before commencing a procedure, replied: 'wash your hands'. This was not the anticipated answer; the answer required was 'explain to the patient'. The students demonstrated a perception of nursing that was dominated by the features of a task and not by the socio-emotional needs of a patient.

It has earlier been identified that the only way in which student nurses could learn communication behaviour was by use of role models, and that the first role model they encountered was the nurse teacher. It could reasonably be expected that she would exhibit 'ideal' communication behaviour as she is usually seen as an ideal practitioner of nursing care. In the event nurse teachers presented as negative role models for communication behaviour. This finding must be regarded as extremely disturbing, especially in view of the fact that nurse learners may choose to copy their behaviour. One is prompted to ask why nurse teachers exhibited the communication behaviour documented.

One explanation is provided by the milieu of nursing education. Teachers themselves may see the environment as artificial and may feel foolish role playing or speaking to a doll. Another explanation relies on the nature of the tasks to be taught. Many tasks are complicated and technical and so a teacher may concentrate on teaching the components of a task without relating the task to the patient with whom it is to be enacted. A further explanation may be that teachers do not regard communication skills as (a) something which needs to be taught (the implication being that we all possess them), or (b) something which can be taught; people either possess them or they do not. A final explanation could be that teachers rarely become involved with patients. They may thus fail to appreciate the importance of communication skills. This latter view seems unlikely. All teachers seemed aware (theoretically) of the value of communication. What they did not seem aware of was that they were not doing anything to ensure that learners became, or remained, good communicators.

In view of their lack of training in communication skills, and the negative examples presented to them by nurse teachers, it is not surprising that the communication behaviour of the student nurse observed was so limited. The communication behaviours of student nurses was found to be uniform across all three hospitals and only 15 per cent of the communications observed (from a total of 1300) were found to be facilitative to the communication process. When one considers that communication behaviours were obtained from thirty-two different student nurse subjects, working in sixteen wards in the three hospitals, this must be regarded as a very disturbing finding.

It is, again, not surprising that the majority of communications provided by nurses were functional, and that, as well as controlling content, nurses also controlled duration (over 90 per cent of interactions being concluded by the nurse). To have allowed social communications and patient control would have demanded levels of communication skill which students did not possess and so, it is argued, they prevented these communications from occurring. It is interesting, however, that when asked at interview which type of communication patients preferred the majority of nurses said 'social'. This is also what patients themselves said, when questioned.

As communication skill development was not a planned part of student nurses' learning experiences, however, it is possible that they may have failed to recognise it as a nursing skill. A significant difference between occupational levels was found in relation to whether or not nurses felt that they had sufficient time to talk to patients, with students alone saying that they usually had enough time to talk to patients. The majority, however, stated that they found it difficult to understand patients' emotions and behaviour, and said that they had been helped to do so by neither school nor ward staff.

Several students at interview exhibited extreme anxiety in relation to this aspect of their work and, when questioned about teaching in interpersonal skills, tended to see acquisition of the skill as capable of reducing their own (rather than patient) discomfort. A student at hospital three said: 'I find it very difficult, it still frightens me', and another said: 'I don't know what to do, I try to avoid these situations'. A student at hospital two was very concerned about her own emotions with regard to patient behaviour:

It bothers me, especially when someone is desperate to talk and you haven't got the time – (long pause), I feel ever so hard, a lot of the patients I don't really like, know what I mean? A lot of the patients you can become very attached to. Perhaps it's the ward that I'm on, you can't really have a conversation. I'm not really convinced that we're doing the right thing anyway, like Mrs. Y with two legs off, I sometimes feel that she's right, she *would* be better gone. There's another lady she tries to tell you something and I can't understand her. I haven't really got the time anyway. If you think what's going on in her mind, she must be absolutely — to put myself in her position . . . I don't really feel for her like I should, to me she's a high carbohydrate diet.

She then went on to rationalise her emotions by saying: 'I care enough to want to do the job in the first place, but you can't have a personal relationship with every patient'.

That nurses did not feel able to cope with patients' emotions may have been recognised by some patients, over half of whom stated that they had felt worried or afraid whilst in hospital (24). Half of this group (13) had not voiced their fears to anyone. They were similarly reticent to ask for things that they might need or want. If a need was not concerned with treatment or care, it was often not seen as legitimate. The majority of patients (28) said that they had not had as many opportunities to talk with nurses as they would have liked, but tended to believe that talking could only occur when nurses had all their (legitimate) 'work' done. A smaller number of patients (7) felt that they had been given insufficient information by nurses. It would seem, from these responses, that patients, as well as nurses, quickly learn that communications between nurses and patients are not valued by the institution within which they are housed. A need existed, but this need was not realised in practice by nurses, although it was recognised in theory.

It is possible that patients do not threaten nurses with informational demands because they realise that to do so would threaten a nurse's 'face'. Goffman (1967) says:

Much of the activity occurring during an encounter can be understood as an effort on everyone's part to get through the occasion and all the unanticipated and unintentional events that can cast participants in an undesirable light, without disrupting the relationship of the participants . . . It seems to be a characteristic of many social relationships that each of the members guarantees to support a given face for the other members in a given situation. To prevent disrup-

tion of these relationships, it is therefore necessary for each member
to avoid destroying the other's face.

It seems that patients recognise that, if they are to succeed in hospital,
they must take on a 'good patient' role. This role prevents them challenging the agents of the institution.

Patients were more frank when asked which skills a junior nurse
should possess, the majority naming skills which could be classed as
interpersonal. Patients believed nurses needed to know 'how to put
people at ease', and 'how to deal with all sorts of people'. Some
patients said that interpersonal skill would lead to better understanding
between patients and nurses. When questioned about methods of nursing care delivery, patients most frequently chose patient, rather than
task allocation, as they said that it would enable them to get to know
the nurses better, and that they would know who to ask if they needed
anything. Patients thus clearly demonstrated a need to communicate
with nurses, nurses recognised this need, but did not meet it. Student
nurses may have failed to meet the need because they felt unable to do
so (they had not been prepared in the skill) or because, unlike senior
nurses, they had not yet learnt to pay lip service to the ideal of communicating with patients. Their view may have been influenced by their
view of what a nurse should do (demonstrate practical nursing skills)
and of which skills are valued by the institution (practical nursing
skills).

Summary

That nurse teachers failed to prepare student nurses for their job on the
ward has been demonstrated and discussed.

Students were not allowed to become proficient in the performance
of practical skills in school, yet they were expected to be proficient
in these skills in the workplace. Nurse teachers may have included
some skills in the curriculum as they recognise that the skills are
commonly demanded in the workplace. To include them, but not to
allow proficiency to develop, creates student anxiety which is compounded when students are expected to perform the skills on the
wards.

The majority of the teaching was provided in nurse training schools,
not clinical areas. It is now generally recognised that the ward is the
most influential learning environment, and that the trained nurse is the

most effective teacher (Wyatt, 1978; Orton, 1980; Fretwell, 1981). On very few occasions (6) were trained nurses used as a teaching resource by nurse teachers. It now seems clear that the nurse teacher's role must change from that of 'expert' to that of facilitator. She cannot, herself, be expected to know all the answers to student learning needs, indeed she may not, if she continues to operate in the isolation of the nurse training school, be aware of many of the student's learning needs. This seems to have been recognised by learners and by service nurses for many years, but not actively by nurse teachers, who continue to try to teach most (if not all) subjects in the syllabus themselves and to do so in schools of nursing.

It has been suggested that nurse teachers may teach 'ideal' rather than 'real' care. It has been alleged (by some service nurses) that this is because nurse teachers do not know what 'real' care comprises (being rather clinically out-of-date or unaware of resource constraints). A move from the classroom to the ward and a change of role from controller of knowledge to facilitator of knowledge would greatly improve other nurses' perceptions of the value of nurse teachers. It has been argued that nurse teachers have a major contribution to make towards setting and maintaining standards of nursing care. They cannot do this unless they teach and learn in the areas of which nursing care is provided.

In addition to feeling inadequately prepared in practical nursing skills, students also felt inadequately prepared in communication skills. It has been argued that nursing is a social profession and that the ability to communicate with patients is fundamental to the art of nursing. None of the three training schools observed prepared students in this skill. Both patients and students expressed the belief that student nurses should be taught communication skills. By failing to meet this need nurse teachers did not prepare student nurses for their role as a nurse.

There are indications that the need for preparation in social skills will become more urgent in the immediate future. Systems of nursing care are changing from task assignment to patient allocation. This demands deeper and closer relationships between nurses and patients than they have at present. Some patients may use this relationship to reduce their own stress (provoked by anxiety). Indications are that they would choose junior learners as those with whom to relate; (patient, hospital two) 'The younger ones seem less experienced at keeping their mouth shut, so you can get more information that way'.

Note

1. Much of the research discussed in this chapter was conducted while the author was a DHSS Nursing Research Fellow.
2. This finding is in line with findings arising from a study of standards of care in four Thames regions (1978) published in *Nursing Times*, 8 June 1978 (p. 944). The majority of nurses sampled (108) said that washing after toilet was 'infrequent or not encouraged'.

References

Abdel-Al, A.H. 'Relating Education to Practice Within a Nursing Context', Unpublished PhD thesis, University of Edinburgh, 1975

Anderson, E. (1973) *The Role of the Nurse*, Royal College of Nursing, London

Annual Report of the Health Service Commissioners (1978-1979), HMSO, London

Armitage, S. (1980) 'Non-compliant recipients of health care', *Nursing Times* Occasional Paper 76, no. 1

Bendall, E. (1975) *So You Passed Nurse*, Royal College of Nursing, London

Birch, J. (1975) *To Nurse or Not to Nurse*, Royal College of Nursing, London

Birch, J. (1979) 'The Anxious Learners', *Nursing Mirror, 148*, 8 February 1979, 17-22

Brown, M. (1977) 'Nursing research; delights and difficulties', *73*, Occasional Paper, *Nursing Times*, 14 July 1977

Carstairs, V. (1970) *Channels of Communication*, Scottish Home and Health Department

Cassee, E.T. (1975) 'Therapeutic behaviour, hospital culture and communication' in Cox, C. and Mead A. (eds.), *A Sociology of Medical Practice*, Collier Macmillan, London

Danzinger, K. (1976) *Interpersonal Communication*, Pergamon Press, Oxford

Dodd, A.P. (1974) 'Towards an Understanding of Nursing', Unpublished PhD thesis, University of London

Faulkner, A. (1981) 'The communicator as a person', *Nursing*, 27 July 1981, 1162-3

Fretwell, J. (1980) 'An inquiry into the ward learning environment', *Nursing Times, 76*, Occasional Paper 26 June 1980

Goffman, E. (1967) *Interaction Ritual*, Penguin London

Gregory, J. (1979) 'Report for the Office of Population Census and Surveys', Published in Royal Commission on the National Health Service, HMSO, London

Hunt, J. (1974) *The Teaching and Practice of Surgical Dressings in Three Hospitals*, Royal College of Nursing, London

Hunt, J. (1981) 'Indicators for nursing practice: the use of research findings', *Journal of Advanced Nursing, 6*, 189-94

Kramer, M. (1974) *Reality Shock: Why Nurses Leave Nursing*, St Louis, C.V. Mosby Co.

McGhee, A. (1961) *The Patient's Attitude to Nursing Care*, E.S. Livingstone, Edinburgh

McIntosh, J. (1977) *Communication and Awareness in a Cancer Ward*, Croom Helm, London; Prodist, New York

Menzies, I. (1970) *The Functioning of Social Systems as a Defence Against Anxiety*, Tavistock Institute of Human Relations

Orton, H. (1981) 'Ward learning climate and student nurse response', *Nursing Times, 77*, Occasional Paper, 4 June 1981

Pepper, R. (1977) Professionalism, Training and Work, PhD thesis, University of Kent
Quenzer, R. (1974) 'The Development of Patient Centred Behaviour Patterns in Nurse Training', Unpublished M.Ed. thesis, University of Manchester
Report of the Committee of Nursing (1972) HMSO, London

Part Three

TEACHING AND INFORMATION SUPPORT SYSTEMS

INTRODUCTION

Bryn D. Davis

As has been shown in the first two parts of this book, various people influence the nurse learner. This final part is concerned with the education of teachers, and the preparation and support of administrators, teachers and clinical staff in their professional and educational roles.

In Chapter 7, Sheahan offers a brief discussion of the nature of teaching, and, from the literature, of ways of studying the teaching process. The importance of personality, attitudes and values is stressed. This reflects the findings of the studies reported in the first two parts of this book.

Those involved in the educational process, as significant others, must, as well as being adequately prepared, also make regular reference to the latest literature, if their practice is to be suitable as an example to the learner and if it is to provide the best care for the patient. In Chapter 8, Wells describes a survey of the kind of reading done by managers, teachers and ward sisters, and of the implementation of research findings in ward practice. Evidence of the minimal amounts of reading and implementation found by Wells is confirmed by Chakrabarty in Chapter 9. Her survey to assess the library and information provision for nurses found very limited resources available for trained staff.

Chakrabarty also describes an attempt to improve the facilities, a theme which is taken up by Bond in the last chapter, where she describes two ways of improving the distribution of information resources to the practitioners in the field.

7 EDUCATING FOR TEACHING NURSING

John Sheahan

Introduction

In this chapter it is intended to provide a brief characterisation of the nature of teaching. Ways of analysing the teaching process are outlined. Specific reference is made to studies relating to personality, attitudes and values. Finally, some signposts are provided for further research.

The Nature of Teaching

When discussing teaching generally, Thompson (1972) suggests that no particular place is required for the activity nor is any professional qualification. He goes on to assert that the greater part of the teaching of young children is undertaken by their parents, and he concludes that teaching is the intention to secure learning on the part of those taught.

Hirst (1971), a leading educational philosopher, has made a thorough analysis of the concept of teaching. He depicts a situation where a teacher opens a window to improve ventilation, sharpens a few pencils, and prevents a squabble between two pupils. All these activities may be accepted as legitimate elements in the teaching process. Hirst goes on to argue that if the teacher did nothing except opening windows, sharpening pencils and so on, no actual teaching would take place. He therefore differentiates between teaching and the extraneous activities just mentioned, and concludes that teaching implies the intention to bring about learning.

Two points emerge from what has been said so far: the first concerns the relationship between teaching and learning, and the second concerns the intuitive element in the teaching and learning process.

Both of the sources cited above included the concept of learning in their characterisations of teaching. In fact Hirst (1971) suggests that the concept of teaching is entirely parasitic on that of learning. It follows from this that any analysis of teaching must take account of the concept of learning.

Underwood (1966) suggests that learning is something we infer to have occurred by observing changes in performance. Thus, we do not observe learning directly. We measure a subject's performance, and if this performance shows certain characteristics, we say that learning has occurred. Learning is therefore a construct, or an intervening variable, which links performance changes and practice.

An alternative definition of learning is offered by Tomlinson (1981), who rightly makes the point that learning tends to be defined in varying ways according to the theoretical standpoint of the person offering the definition. According to this source tendencies change as a result of action or experience. Tomlinson goes on to elaborate on his definition. In his formulation capacities correspond to cognitive learning expressed in terms of knowing how to do something. Tendencies correspond to motivational learning and are expressed in terms of preferences and values, that is, tendencies to act, react, think, judge and so on.

This account of learning is intentionally brief since its purpose is to remind us that we need to take learning into account in any characterisation of teaching. Tomlinson (1971) can be recommended as a good source for up-to-date references to research on teaching and learning. A variety of viewpoints relating to learning will be found in Ausubel, Novak and Hanesian (1978), Borger and Seaborne (1966), Deese and Hulse (1967), Gagne (1977), Hilgard (1964), Howe (1980) and Lindsay and Norman (1977).

It is likely that few of us have not learned important lessons from people who would make no claim to be teachers, such as parents, guardians or other significant people in our lives. If this is so, then it might be argued that since intuitive approaches to teaching can be successful, we could leave it at that. There is no doubt that intuition is an important element in our lives and there is no suggestion that it should be otherwise. However, it is the case that practices based on intuition alone are unlikely to be predictable. It is also the case that we like to be able to predict the consequences of our actions and this is where theory comes in.

To have a theory about anything is to have an explanation for it. To achieve that is the goal of science, and a discipline has no theory until it has a coherent explanation for the things it studies. The common view is that theory is abstract, difficult and detached from both reality and practice. Yet it might be argued that there is nothing as practical as a good theory since we can use it to both explain and predict and thus avoid shooting in the dark.

An ideal approach to teaching would take account of both intuitive insights and scientific theory in a balanced way. There are however some obstacles in the way of achieving this ideal. Cohen (1976) writes of traditionalism, of the notion that teaching cannot be taught and of the mystique of teaching. Bruner (1966), who formulated a theory of instruction, acknowledges that his theory is not without its weaknesses. In a review of research into teaching methods in higher education Beard, Bligh and Harding (1978) concluded that we seem as far as ever from developing a theory of instruction. However, they add that there is a fairly substantial body of information to provide ideas for teachers who wish to try new methods. Beard *et al*. (1978) can be recommended as a useful source relating to research on teaching; over 500 references are cited and are reviewed in a succinct yet critical manner. The following sources deal with aspects of teacher education: Allen (1963), Dunkerton (1981), Gibson (1972), Hogben (1979), Rousseau (1978), Nias (1977), Stones and Morris (1972).

The Teaching Process

Teaching is a paradoxical activity. At one level it is something that anyone can do, yet at another level it can be characterised as a complex activity involving intellectual and social interaction which makes use of concepts from philosophy, psychology and sociology. What follows are some approaches for analysing the process of teaching.

In the first instance the work of Lewin (1935) will be considered. In Lewin's view human behaviour (B) is a function (F) of the person (P) and the environment (E) in which the person finds himself. The relationship has been expressed as an equation as follows, $B = f(P.E)$. In the table that follows (Table 7.1), some of the elements which comprise each part of Lewin's equation are set out together with a reference to the literature in each case.

Since teaching is the intention to bring about learning, the behaviour which is of concern to the teacher is, of course, learning. In fact it is common to express the intended outcomes of teaching as behavioural objectives, that is, what it is the learner will be able to do at the end of a learning experience. These are generally expressed as the cognitive, affective and psychomotor domains of learning. In Table 7.1 social, moral and experiential domains have been added to make a more comprehensive analysis of the teaching process. It is argued that learning takes place in a social context, it is a value-laden activity and it involves the reorganisation and integration of experience on the part of the learner. If it is accepted that this is the case, then the social, moral and experiential aspects ought to be taken into account in analysing the teaching process.

Table 7.1: A modified version of Lewin's (1935) analysis of human behaviour adapted to an educational context

Behaviour Learning	Person	Environment
Cognitive (Bloom, 1956)	Biological (Pugh, 1978)	Attitudes (Elms, 1976)
Affective (Krathwohl *et al.*, 1964)	Intelligence (Butcher, 1968)	Expectations (Nash, 1976)
Psychomotor (Harrow, 1972)	Memory (Herriott, 1974)	Groups (Shaw, 1976)
Social (Bandura and Walters 1963)	Motivation (Lunzer, 1968)	
Moral (Niblett, 1963)	Perception (Vernon, 1970)	Role (Sheahan, 1981)
Experiential (Boydell, 1976)	Personality (Fontana, 1977)	Social climate (White and Jippitt, 1960)
	Self Concept (Burns, 1977)	Teachers (Morrison and McIntyre, 1973)
	Thinking (Burton and Radford, 1978)	Teacher/learner relations (Hargreaves, 1972)

Stating the learning objectives is a necessary but not a sufficient condition to bring about learning, account needs to be taken of factors which relate to the person. It might be argued that a level of intelligence appropriate to the learning task is an obvious condition for learning to take place. But there is also the will to learn or motivational factors. Lack of motivation may result in an intelligent brain not being used to its full potential. Motivational factors may relate to the underlying personality; introverts are said to be more at home with academic study than extroverts and this has been related to their biological make-up (Eysenck, 1967). Academic success or otherwise may be explained in relation to the personality traits of the learner, but this is not the only explanation possible, there is also the self concept of the person. (Burns (1977) provides a useful review of the self concept in relation to education, and Purkey (1970) concluded that there was a significant relationship between the self concept and academic achievement.) The pattern of perceptual organisation, the style of thinking and the ability to memorise are all related to how well a person learns and therefore need to be taken into account, but so must the social context in which learning takes place.

At a general level the ethos or the tone of the educational setting may be influenced by, for example, the self-attitudes of the teachers, their expectations of the learners and their attitudes to teaching approaches, such as formal or informal methods. Morrison and McIntyre (1973, 1975) and Hargreaves (1972) provide useful analyses of the social aspects of education.

The significance of teacher expectations in the educational process has been a subject of much interest since the publication of Rosenthal and Jacobson's (1968) study. This study has been heavily criticised on methodological grounds and replicate studies have come to different conclusions. However, interest in the subject remains and Nash (1976) provides a useful review of the research which has been done.

Expectations are sometimes known as self-fulfilling prophesies and the following elements are thought to be involved in the process. In the first place, and for a variety of reasons, the teacher expects specific behaviour and achievement from particular learners. Because of these different expectations, the teacher behaves differently towards them. This treatment tells the learner what behaviour and achievement the teacher expects. This in turn may affect the learner's self-concept, achievement motivation and level of aspiration. High expectation learners will be led to achieve at high levels, the converse being true for the low-expectation learner. The words 'may affect' have to be included because the evidence relating to teacher expectations is far from conclusive.

The concept of role is an important factor in social relations. It has been defined by Kelvin (1973) who writes 'very simply, a role consists of the functions of the individual who assumes it'. There are a number of aspects to role. The term 'enacted role' refers to the behaviour displayed by an individual in a particular position within an organisation, for example, a nurse learner or a nurse tutor. The perceived role is defined as the perception of the behaviour associated with a certain position, again it might be a nurse learner or a nurse tutor. The expected role is defined as the set of expectations held by group members for the behaviour of one in a particular position in the group. Nurse tutors will have a set of expectations and conversely nurse learners. A related concept is that of predicted role which refers to expectations based on probabilities which are derived from the expectation that a number will continue to behave as in the past, for example, punctual/unpunctual, tidy/untidy, conscientious/careless. Lastly, there is what is called the prescribed role. This designates the expectations related to the regulative forms of a group, representing expectations as to what one in a particular position ought to do.

Mismatches between role enactment and role perception and different expectations relating to role predictions and role prescriptions interact in various combinations to give rise to role confusion and role conflict. In education these are likely to impinge upon the teaching and learning process. In a study of the nurse tutor's role (Sheahan, 1981), using the statistical technique of factor analysis, twelve factors were identified. When nurse teachers and nurse learners were compared in relation to these factors, agreement was found between the two groups in relation to four factors, but there was disagreement in relation to the eight remaining. It would be unwise to come to any firm conclusions on the basis of one study, but it does seem to be an area worthy of further research.

Another significant dimension in the teaching and learning process is the social climate in which it is conducted. White and Lippitt (1960) describe three social climates, which are authoritarian, democratic and laissez-faire. The conclusion seems to be that a democratic set up can be efficient. Work-motivation appears to be stronger and such conditions are also more conducive to originality.

From what has been outlined above, Levin's modified BPE approach provides a useful model for analysing the teaching and learning process, and the aspects covered are meant to be representative rather than comprehensive in nature. There are however alternative ways of looking at teaching and learning and two will be considered now.

Cronbach and Snow (1977) formulated an aptitude-treatment interaction model which is abbreviated to ATIs. The aptitude element takes account of the learner's ability, with the emphasis on intelligence and personality factors. The so called treatment interactions take account of the teaching and learning strategies used and the context of the educational activity. There are similarities between the BPE and the ATI approach; but the ATI approach places more emphasis on intelligence, whereas the BPE approach allows for a more wide-ranging analysis of the teaching and learning process.

Whether a BPE or an ATI approach is used in the analysis of the educational process, what emerges is the great variety of individual differences among the learners. Making a thorough analysis of the factors involved is one thing, but incorporating these in terms of practical proposals for teaching is another matter. This is where the concept of matching models in education comes in. Hunt (1971) has given his attention to this subject. The rationale for the matching models approach is that every learner is different. From this, as the sub-title of

Hunt's (1971) book suggests (the coordination of teaching methods with student characteristics) the aim is to match the learner and the teaching and learning strategy, in other words to individualise the process of education.

The constraints of space allow for no more than a thumbnail sketch of the matching models approach. However it may be of interest to nurse educationalists who deal with the nursing process which, of course, in essence is individualised nursing care. If there is a case for individualised nursing care, there may also be a case for individualised education for the learner; or at least an individualised element, for one has to take account of the ratio of nurse teachers to nurse learners.

For teachers of nursing, whether committed to the BPE model or not, there is an increasing volume of research to draw on and to illuminate their approach to teaching and learning. The evidence is to be found in the present volume: Part one deals mostly with the person element of the BPE models in relation to nurse learners; Part two deals with elements mostly in the environment. However, as well as taking account of the characteristics of the learners, account also needs to be taken of the characteristics of the teachers involved. What follows are accounts of research relating to the personality traits, the social attitudes and the values of teachers of nursing.

Personality

In a review article Lewis and Cooper (1976) cite 60 references relating to the personalities of young nurses. The evidence emerging is mixed; some studies suggest that personality assessments are good predictors, other studies suggest poor predictive powers for such assessments. There appears to be less evidence relating to the personality profiles of senior nurses. An exception is the study by Cooper, Lewis and Moores (1976), who used Cattell's Sixteen Personality Factor (16PF) Questionnaire (Cattell, Eber and Tatuoka, 1970) and found that the personality profiles of a sample of senior nurses were substantially different from those of student nurses.

A study by Sheahan (1980), also using 16PF, came to a similar conclusion. The size of the sample was 124 and comprised full-time student teachers of nursing (n = 30), first year part-time student teachers of nursing (n = 22), second year part-time student teachers of nursing (n = 26), and nurses attending first line management courses (n = 46) and now called 'managers'. The overall conclusion was that the profiles of the subjects were more homogeneous than hetrogeneous. Significant differences were found between the managers and the second year part-time teachers on Factor H (shy-venturesome), and on Factor Q2 (group dependent-self sufficient). The teachers were found to be more venturesome and self-sufficient than the managers. Apart from these differences the profiles of the subjects were to be found principally within the average band of the 16PF profile except that all groups were found to be more intelligent than average. The managers tended to be more reserved, more trusting and more group-dependent than average. The teachers tended to be more self-sufficient and forthright than average.

When the findings of this study were compared with the findings of other studies relating to the personalities of nurses, it appears that senior nurses have different and more stable profiles than young student nurses.

Attitudes

In defining attitudes Elms (1976) makes the point that an individual will have positive or negative feelings about many of the things in which he believes and suggests that these positive and negative feelings about the objects in his psychological world are his attitudes. No doubt there are many examples of positive attitudes in nursing, but there is also evidence of negative ones. Towell (1975) showed that many nurses adopt impersonal attitudes towards patients and Stockwell (1972) comes to a similar conclusion. Studies by House and Sims (1976) and by Sims (1976) dealt with aspects of the attitudes of nurse teachers to their jobs. Studies such as those cited need to be taken into account when analysing the process of teaching and learning nursing. However, there is also a case for taking into account the attitudes of nurse teachers to teaching.

In general education there is a considerable body of evidence relating to the attitudes of teachers and the studies by Butcher (1968) and McIntyre and Morrison (1967) are cited as examples. These studies relate to the work of Oliver (1953) and Oliver and Butcher (1962), and as a consequence Oliver (1969) constructed his Survey of Opinions about Education questionnaire, which Sheahan (1980) used in conjunction with the 16PF study reported above.

The Oliver (1969) questionnaire is in three sections. The first is a measure of tender-mindedness (T) and comprises 14 items; the middle section is a measure of radicalism (R) and comprises 12 items; the remaining section is a measure of naturalism (N) and comprises 10 items (naturalism embodies a subject centredness—pupil centredness dichotomy). Split half reliabilities for the questionnaire are reported as $n = 0.73$, $R = 0.84$, $T = 0.84$.

When the data from this study were analysed significant differences were found in relation to radicalism between the managers and the full-time student teachers; between the managers and the first-year part-time student teachers on tender-mindedness; and between the second-year part-time teachers also on tender-mindedness. The teachers in the study were more tender-minded than the managers and one group was found to be more radical. Apart from these differences the social attitudes of the various sub-groups showed a good deal of similarity. On naturalism, for example, no significant differences were found between the mean scores of any of the sub-groups and the direction of the attitude was toward person-centredness.

Does one teach a subject or people? This is the type of question which leads to a chicken and egg type of argument for clearly both elements are involved in the teaching and learning process. Perhaps the question should be about where the emphasis is put. The evidence from this study suggests that slightly more emphasis is put on the people. Perhaps this is not surprising since nursing is, among other things, about caring for people. And nurse tutors may be expected to retain this attribute.

Values

Whether a teacher emphasises the subject matter or the person in the process of teaching can be explained in terms of attitudes, but it is also possible to offer explanations in relation to the concept of values. Milton Rokeach has made a lifetime study of human values and examples of his works are available (Rokeach 1960, 1967, 1970, 1973).

Rokeach (1973) defines a value as an enduring belief that a specific mode of conduct or end-state of existence is personally or socially preferable to an opposite mode of conduct or end-state of existence. The modes of conduct he calls instrumental values, and these are sub-divided into moral values (courage, helpfulness, honesty, politeness) and competence values (capable, logical, responsible, self-controlled). End-states of existence are called terminal values and these are also of two sorts. One category includes personal values such as happiness, inner harmony, pleasure, salvation; the other category includes social values such as equality, freedom, national security, world peace and so on.

Sheahan (1980a) used Rokeach's Survey of Values with a group of nurse tutor students (n = 32). This questionnaire comprises 18 instrumental values statements (some examples of the items are given above) and 18 terminal value statements (some examples are also given above). A ranking scale is used; the respondents are asked to rank the value that is most important to them as number one and so on until all the items are ranked.

In Sheahan (1980b) the Study of Values questionnaire was set at the beginning and end of a nurse tutor's course. When an appropriate statistical test was applied to the data the differences between the before and after rankings of the value statements were very few, indicating perhaps that, as asserted in the definition, values are enduring beliefs.

Nursing and the teaching of nursing is a value-laden activity and while there is an emerging literature of the subject, for example, Meyer (1960), O'Neill (1973), Garvin (1976), Rhodes (1977), Colling (1980), Schröck (1980), it appears that this area of nursing education is ripe for further research.

Further Research

Education for what? This is a question worthy of the attention of every educator and the answers are likely to be of a diverse nature. However, it is conceivable that the transmission and the creation of knowledge are likely to be well represented among the answers. The process of teaching, among other things, involves the transmission of knowledge. It is through research that knowledge is created.

Too often and too strongly does mere opinion hold the field instead of information gathered from observation and experiment. Studies relating to nurse tutors appear to be few in number. Clarke (1977) in a review of research in nurse education cites only four studies and these were Dutton (1968), Lancaster (1972), General Nursing Council (1975) and Gannon (1975). In the present chapter it has been necessary to draw heavily on the research findings in general education because examples relating to nursing education did not always exist. This means, of course, that there is plenty of scope for further research.

Reference to Table 7.1 suggests three broad areas which could be usefully explored through further research. The behaviour element could be extended to take account of how changes in behaviour (learning) are brought about. Questions such as why, what, how, who, when and where suggest themselves. These are pedagogical questions or perhaps more accurately androgogical questions (Knowles, 1970) since in nursing education we are dealing with adults. In relation to the person element there is scope, for example, to study aspects of motivation, perception, personality and the self concept. Similarly, in relation to the environment topics such as expectations, role, social climate and teacher/learner relations are also ripe for further study.

There is a wealth of literature relating to research methods in education. The works of Gage (1963), Tuckman (1972), Kerlinger (1973), Travers (1973, 1978), and Cohen and Manion (1980) are but a few examples. Another useful book is that by Cohen (1976). As its subtitle suggests, it is a manual of materials and methods which might be used in educational research. It is, of course, written for researchers in general education, but it is likely that some of the approaches could be modified for use in nursing education. However, books on research methods are only helpful up to a point; the best way to learn about research is to actually do it.

References

Allen, E.A. (1963) 'Professional training of teachers: a review of research,' *Educational Research, 5*, 200-15

Ausubel, D.P., Novak, J.D. and Hanesian, H. (1978) *Educational Psychology: A Cognitive View* 2nd edn, Holt, Rinehart & Winston, New York

Bandura, A. and Walters, R. (1963) *Social Learning and Personality Development*, Holt, Rinehart & Winston, New York

Beard, R.M., Bligh, D.A. and Harding, A.G. (1978) *Research into Teaching Methods in Higher Education* 4th edn, Society for Research into Higher Education, Guildford

Bloom, B.S. (ed.) (1956) *Taxonomy of Educational Objectives: Cognitive Domain*, Longman, London

Borger, R. and Seaborne, A.E.M. (1966) *The Psychology of Learning*, Penguin, Harmondsworth

Boydell, T. (1976) *Experiential Learning*, Manchester Monographs 5, Manchester University Press

Bruner, J.S. (1966) *Towards a Theory of Instruction*, Norton, New York

Burns, R.B. (1977) 'The self concept and its relevance to academic achievement' in Child, D. (ed.), *Readings in Psychology for the Teacher*, Holt, Rinehart and Winston, London

Burton, A. and Radford, J. (eds.) (1978) *Thinking in Perspective: Critical Essays in the Study of Thought Processes*, Methuen, London

Butcher, H.J. (1965) 'The attitudes of student teachers to education,' *British Journal of Social and Clinical Psychology, 4*, 17-24

Butcher, H.J. (1968) *Human Intelligence: its Nature and Assessment*, Methuen, London

Cattell, R.B., Eber, H.W. and Tatuoka, M.M. (1970) *Handbook for the Sixteen Personality Factor Questionnaire (16PF)*, NFER, Slough

Clarke, M. (1977) 'Research in nurse education,' *Nursing Times* Occasional Papers *73*, 25-8

Cohen, L. (1976) *Educational Research in Classrooms and Schools: a manual of materials and methods*. Harper & Row, London

Cohen, L. and Manion, L. (1977) *A Guide to Teaching Practice*, Methuen, London

Cohen, L. and Manion, L. (1980) *Research Methods in Education*, Croom Helm, London

Colling, J. (1980) 'The expected occupational satisfactions of student nurses,' *Nursing Times, 76*, (23 October) 1896-8

Cooper, C.L., Lewis, B.L. and Moores, B. (1976) 'Personality profiles of long serving senior nurses: implications for recruitment and selection,' *International Journal of Nursing Studies, 13*, 251-7

Cronbach, L.J. and Snow, R.E. (1977) *Aptitudes and Instructional Methods: A Handbook for Research on Interaction*, Irvington, New York

Deese, J. and Hulse, S.H. (1967) *The Psychology of Learning*, McGraw-Hill, New York

Dunkerton, J. (1981) 'Should classroom observations be quantitative?' *Educational Research, 23*, 144-51

Dutton, A. (1968) *Factors Affecting Recruitment of Nurse Tutors*, King Edward's Hospital Fund, London

Elms, A.C. (1976) *Attitudes*. Open University Press, Milton Keynes

Eysenck, H.J. (1967) *The Biological Basis of Personality*, Thomas, Springfield, Illinois

Fontana, D. (1977) *Personality and Education*, Open Books, London

Gage, N. (ed.) (1963) *Handbook of Research on Teaching*, Rand McNally, Chicago

Gagne, R.M. (1977) *The Conditions of Learning*, 3rd edn, Holt, Rinehart and Winston, New York

Gannon, B. (1975) 'Predicting success in clinical teacher students.' *Nursing Times* Occasional Paper *71*, 33-5 (17 April)

Garvin, B.J. (1976) 'Values of male nursing students', *Nursing Research, 25*, 352-7

General Nursing Council for England and Wales (1975) *Teachers of Nursing 102* General Nursing Council, London

Gibson, D.R. (1972) 'Professional socialisation: the effects of a college course upon role-conceptions of students in teacher training,' *Educational Research, 14*, 213-19

Hargreaves, D.H. (1972) *Interpersonal Relations in Education*, Routledge and Kegan Paul, London

Harrow, A.S. (1972) *A Taxonomy of the Psychomotor Domain: a guide for developing behavioural objectives*. McKay, New York

Herriott, P. (1974) *Attributes of Memory*, Methuen, London

Hilgard, E.R. (ed.) (1964) *Theories of Learning and Instruction*, National Society for the Study of Education, Chicago

Hirst, P.H. (1971) 'What is teaching?' in Peters, R.S. (ed.) (1973) *The Philosophy of Education*, Oxford University Press, Oxford

Hogben, D. (1979) 'Early changes in teacher attitude,' *Educational Research, 21*, 212-19

House, V. and Sims, A. (1976) 'Teachers of nursing in the United Kingdom: a description of their attitudes,' *Journal of Advanced Nursing, 1*, 495-505

Howe, M.J.A. (1980) *The Psychology of Human Learning*, Harper and Row, London

Hunt, D.E. (1971) *Matching Models in Education: the coordination of teaching methods with student characteristics*. Monograph Series No. 10. Ontario Institute for Studies in Education, Ontario

Kelvin, P. (1973) *The Bases of Social Behaviour: An Approach in Terms of Order and Value*, Holt, Rinehart and Winston, London

Kerlinger, F.N. (1973) *Review of Research in Education*, Peacock, Itasca, Illinois

Knowles, M.S. (1970) *The Modern Practice of Adult Education: Androgogy versus Pedagogy*, Association Press, New York

Krathwohl, D.R., Bloom, B.S. and Masia, B.B. (1964) *Taxonomy of Educational Objectives: Affective Domain*, Longman, London

Lancaster, A. (1972) *Nurse Teachers: The Report of an Opinion Survey*, Churchill Livingstone, Edinburgh

Lewin, K. (1935) *A Dynamic Theory of Personality*, McGraw-Hill, New York

Lewis, B.R. and Cooper, C.L. (1976) 'Personality measurement among nurses: a review,' *International Journal of Nursing Studies, 13*, 209-29

Lindsay, P.H. and Norman, D.A. (1977) *Human Information Processing*, 2nd edn, Academic Press, New York

Lunzer, E.A. (1968) *The Regulation of Behaviour*, Staples Press, London

McIntyre, D. and Morrison, A. (1967) 'The educational opinions of teachers in training,' *British Journal of Social and Clinical Psychology, 6*, 32-7

Meyer, G.R. (1960) *Tenderness and Technique: Nursing Values in Transition*, University of California, Los Angeles

Morrison, A. and McIntyre, D. (1973) *Teachers and Teaching*, Penguin, Harmondsworth

Morrison, A. and McIntyre, D. (1975) *Schools and Socialization*, Penguin, Harmondsworth

Nash, R. (1976) *Teacher Expectations and Pupil Learning*, Routledge and Kegan Paul, London

Nias, J. (1977) 'What should Nellie do? Student's role – expectations for head and class teachers on school-supervised practice,' *British Journal of Teacher Education, 3*, 121-30

Niblett, W.R. (1963) *Moral Education in a Changing Society*, Faber and Faber, London

Oliver, R.A.C. (1953) 'Attitudes to education,' *British Journal of Educational Studies, 11*, 31-41

Oliver, R.A.C. (1969) *Survey of Opinions about Education: Notes for Users*, University of Manchester

Oliver, R.A.C. and Butcher, H.J. (1962) 'Teachers' attitudes to education: the structure of educational attitudes,' *British Journal of Social and Clinical Psychology, 1*, 56-69

O'Neill, M.F. (1973) A study of baccalaureate nursing student values. *Nursing Research, 22*, 437-43

Pugh, G.E. (1978) *The Biological Origin of Human Values*, Routledge & Kegan Paul, London

Purkey, W. (1970) *Self Concept and School Achievement*, Prentice Hall, New Jersey

Rhodes, B. (1977) 'The instrumental values of nurses', *Nursing Mirror, 145*, 29-30 (10 November)

Rokeach, M. (1960) *The Open and Closed Mind: investigations into the nature of belief systems and personality systems*, Basic Books, New York

Rokeach, M. (1967) *Value Survey*, Halgren Tests, Sunnyvale, California

Rokeach, M. (1970) *Beliefs, Attitudes and Change*, San Francisco: Jossey Bass

Rokeach, M. (1973) *The Nature of Human Values*, The Free Press, New York

Rosenthal, R. and Jacobson, L. (1968) *Pygmalion in the Classroom*, Holt, Rinehart and Winston, New York

Rousseau, H.J. (1978) 'The impact of educational theory on teachers,' *British Journal of Educational Studies, 36*, 60-71

Schröck, R.A. (1980) 'A question of honesty in nursing practice,' *Journal of Advanced Nursing, 5*, 135-48

Shaw, M.E (1976) *Group Dynamics: the psychology of small group behavior*, 2nd edn, McGraw-Hill, New York

Sheahan, J. (1980a) The personality traits and social attitudes of student teachers of nursing, unpublished MSc dissertation, University of Bradford)

Sheahan, J. (1980b) A pre-course and post-course assessment of the values of nurse tutor students, unpublished

Sheahan, J. (1981) 'A study of the nurse tutor's role,' *Journal of Advanced Nursing, 6*, 125-35

Sheahan, J. (1982) 'The research interests of nurse tutor students,' Occasional Papers. *Nursing Times 78*(5), 17-20

Sims, A. (1976) 'Teachers of nursing in the United Kingdom: some characteristics of teachers and their jobs,' *Journal of Advanced Nursing, 1*, 377-89

Stockwell, F. (1972) *The Unpopular Patient*, Royal College of Nursing, London

Stones, E. and Morris, S. (1972) 'The assessment of practical teaching,' *Educational Research, 14*, 110-19

Thompson, K. (1972) *Education and Philosophy: a practical approach*, Blackwell, Oxford

Tomlinson, P. (1981) *Understanding Teaching: interactive educational psychology*, McGraw-Hill, London

Towell, D. (1975) *Understanding Psychiatric Nursing*, Royal College of Nursing, London

Travers, R.M. (ed.) (1973) *Second Handbook of Research on Teaching: a project of the American Educational Research Association*, Rand McNally, Chicago

Travers, R.M. (1978) *An Introduction to Educational Research*, 4th edn, Macmillan, New York

Tuckman, B.W. (1972) *Conducting Educational Research*, Harcourt Brace Jovanovich, New York

Underwood, B.J. (1966) *Experimental Psychology*, 2nd edn, Appleton-Century-Crofts, New York

Vernon, M.D. (1970) *Perception Through Experience*, Methuen, London

White, R. and Lippitt, R.O. (1960) *Autocracy and Democracy*, Harper and Row, New York

8 A SURVEY OF UPTAKE BY SENIOR NURSING STAFF OF NURSING LITERATURE ON RESEARCH AND EFFECTS ON NURSING PRACTICE

John Wells

In 1980 the author of this chapter undertook a survey of senior nursing staff to ascertain their attitudes to nursing practice research; to sample their behaviour toward nursing practice research – that is, whether they were active in seeking information about research already undertaken and published; and whether they have taken action that would, or had, put this knowledge to work in their own areas of clinical responsibility. The survey was also concerned to find out whether the respondents believed that impediments prevented the utilisation of nursing practice research findings and, if present, what these impediments were perceived to be (Wells, 1980).

The Need for Research-based Practice

Twenty years have passed since Professor J. Brotherston, at a research seminar organised by the International Foundation and held in New Delhi in 1960, emphasised that: 'Whereas the ability and opportunity to carry out research must be limited to a minority in any profession, an urgent and understanding sense of the need for research should be part of the mental equipment of every member of any profession worthy of the name' (Brotherston, 1960). That nursing should be a research-based profession was recognised by the United Kingdom Committee on Nursing (Briggs Committee) in its Report in 1972. Paragraph 370 includes the following, '. . . we consider that it is also necessary to emphasise the need for research.' 'Nor is there enough emphasis on research as a prelude to innovation. Nursing should be a research-based profession.' And, '. . . a sense of the need for research should become part of the mental equipment of every practising nurse and midwife'. Paragraph 377 concerns communication about research. It states, 'The conclusions of research – and in some cases the discussion of research schemes – have been discussed at conferences and during short courses. If research is to lead to innovation, we regard it as essential that nurses and midwives in all parts of the country should be given the opportunity of initiating and participating in such activities' (Briggs Report, 1972).

There are several implications arising from the above. The first is that every nurse should base her nursing practice on rigorously researched and proven methods, principles and theories, that in order to do so research findings must be published in understandable form and that nurses actively search the nursing literature and read published research findings. It also implies that nurses must be able to identify what, if any, elements in published findings are applicable for utilisation in care of patients for whom they have responsibility, and that the right conditions must be created to facilitate research-based practice through education, management support and resource provision.

If it can be assumed that little argument would arise among nurses about these factors, how do nurses act? Do they equip themselves with knowledge of available nursing research findings and put these into nursing practice? The Report of the Royal Commission on the National Health Service (1979) appeared optimistic. In paragraph 13.56, headed Nursing Research, it states, 'There is heartening evidence in the literature and in practice that nurses are beginning to apply research findings in their work, in for example, the prevention of pressure sores, feeding the unconscious patient, the management of pain, and the promotion of continence.' No data are supplied to support this statement. Very little is known about how nurses gain awareness, evaluate and make decisions on the adoption or rejection of innovations in nursing. This researcher was less optimistic than the Royal Commission about the progress being made and believed that the vast majority of nurses are unaware of what nursing practice research findings are available, are ill-equipped to evaluate the potential use of these findings, that few nurses in positions of responsibility read nursing research report findings, and, if they have read them will probably not have acted to change nursing practice.

Survey Design

A survey was designed and carried out in 1980 to try to ascertain what senior nurses were doing to equip themselves with knowledge of nursing practice innovations and whether they had adopted such innovations into clinical areas for which they were responsible (Wells, 1980). The survey was much larger in scope than the subject material contained within this chapter and the following account is, of necessity more limited.

A number of hypotheses were formulated and among them are the following four, shown in Table 8.1.

Table 8.1: Hypotheses for testing

Hypothesis A

Inservice and other post-registration teaching will be found to be absent or inadequate in preparing nurses to evaluate and utilise findings of nursing practice research reports.

Hypothesis B

A general lack of awareness will be found among clinical nurses and nurse managers about nursing practice innovations available in published reports.

Hypothesis C

Nurses do not actively seek out nursing practice research reports and read them.

Hypothesis D

Few wards will be found to have adopted findings of nursing practice research reports.

There were constraints of time and resources that largely governed the scope of the survey and it was decided to collect data by personal interview, using a predetermined interview schedule.

It was taken for granted that the ward sister is in the key role in determining the practice of nursing care, what nursing care is practised and how it is practised. The role of nursing service managers is to provide support by providing resources, information, advice and encouragement, and to formulate nursing policies and monitor their effectiveness. The role of nurse educationalists is to provide support by way of information and the transmission of knowledge and skills. Nursing service managers and nurse educationalists should be 'enablers' and 'facilitators' for clinical nurses. This being so, it was decided to interview ward sisters of adult wards, nurse managers from nursing officer up to divisional nursing officer, and nurse educationalists from clinical teacher up to director of nurse education.

It was thought that there would be little difference between staff in teaching and non-teaching districts, but it was decided to interview in one of each type of district because there would be doubts about possible differences if this was not done. It was decided to choose districts in the Thames regions that the researcher had not worked in or had detailed knowledge of through other connections.

Population Sample

In both districts a list of wards and lists of nurse manager and nurse educationalist role-holders was prepared for the researcher.

In the teaching district the nurses interviewed were twelve ward sisters, five nurse managers and four nurse educationalists. This represents roughly one-fifth of the ward sisters, one quarter of the nursing service managers and one quarter of the nurse educationalists. In the non-teaching district the nurses interviewed were sixteen ward sisters, nine nurse managers and four nurse educationalists. This represents roughly one-quarter of the ward sisters, one-third of nurse managers and nearly one-half of nurse educationalists. It is not possible to have a truly 'representative' or 'average' district regardless of how the districts are chosen. Both were in the Thames regions and these regions may differ from others in different parts of the country. As noted above, one was a teaching and one a non-teaching district.

As neither of the population samples from within the districts were selected randomly, there must be uncertainty as to the generality of the findings. However, considering the combination of factors that brought researcher and respondents together (ie mutual agreement on interview days between researcher and hospital representative, staff holidays, days off, sickness, consultants' rounds and other extremely pressing circumstances which prevented two interviews taking place) it seems unlikely that the population samples could be markedly biased in any particular direction.

The Interviews

The interviews were conducted in a quiet private place. Before each interview, the researcher identified himself as a nurse and postgraduate student at Brunel University. He briefly explained that he was interested in discovering the nature and extent of some of the problems that were hampering the implementation of nursing practice research findings into nursing practice and guaranteed anonymity of each respondent and the district. He then asked if the respondent was willing to answer questions. There were no refusals. In both health districts all staff encountered showed interest and cooperation.

The researcher read the questions out exactly as written in the interview schedule. Very few respondents asked for elaboration or clarification of questions, but the questions concerned were: Q15 ('What do you mean by nursing research appreciation?'), Q26 ('Do you mean only proper research?' 'Do you include students' minor research?' – the latter in the teaching district), Q28 ('What is a Nursing Research Interest Group?').

Results

Ward Sisters

The analysed data from the questionnaires have produced some interesting findings, but space restriction here has meant that only the most relevant data have been included. (The full dissertation can be perused if further detail is required.)

The two district populations of ward sisters were broadly similar but an obvious difference was that those in the teaching district were younger than those in the non-teaching district by a mean-to-mean difference of about 9 years. In the teaching district they have been qualified on average 3.7 years less but have been in the grade slightly longer.

Question numbers refer to question numbers in the main interview schedule (see Wells, 1980).

In the teaching district all twelve wards were used for nurse training. Eleven were acute general, one was a geriatric ward.

In the non-teaching district twelve wards were used for nurse training. Nine were acute general, three were geriatric wards. Three non-teaching wards were geriatric, one was a general ward for minor surgery and subacute conditions.

A number of questions were asked to discover what, if any, preparation the ward sisters had had to equip them for evaluating nursing practice research reports or if they were active in pursuit of further knowledge about research. These questions and the answers obtained are contained in Table 8.2. Following the table questions with answers needing more detailed breakdown are listed. This issue is pursued further in Chapters 9 and 10.

Table 8.2: Questions to ward sisters

		Yes	No
Q10	During your training, did you have sessions on research appreciation?	0	26
Q11	During your training, did you read nursing practice research reports?	0	26
Q12	During your training, was nursing practice taught based on particular nursing practice research reports?	0	26
Q15	Since qualifying, have you attended nursing research appreciation sessions?	0	26
Q20	Have you had any inservice training concerned with evaluating nursing practice research?	0	26
Q22	Have you been offered help to evaluate nursing practice research reports?	0	26
Q24	Have you requested help to evaluate nursing practice research reports?	0	26
Q28	Are you aware of the existence of Nursing Research Interest Groups?		
	(Teaching)	4 (33%)	8 (67%)
	(Non-teaching)	7 (44%)	9 (56%)
Q29	Are you a member of a Nursing Research Interest Group?	0	26
Q30	Has anyone encouraged you to attend a Nursing Research Interest Group?	*2	24

*both from non-teaching district but neither had attended.

Q13. Do you keep up with nursing research practice now?
Teaching District: Yes = 4 (33%); no = 8 (67%)
Non-teaching District: Yes = 6 (37.5%); no = 10 (62.5%)

Q14. If so, how?

In the teaching district eight said that they read *Nursing Times* regularly and two more occasionally. Three read *Nursing Mirror* regularly and three more occasionally. All those who said they read *Nursing Mirror* also read *Nursing Times*. Two said they never read a professional publication. Only two ward sisters read other than *Nursing Times* and *Nursing Mirror*. One had read some RCN research monographs. One had read text books and articles on the nursing process.

In the non-teaching district seven said that they read *Nursing Times* regularly and two more occasionally. Six read *Nursing Mirror* regularly and four more occasionally. Eight read both, but five never read a professional publication. Only three read other than *Nursing Times* and *Nursing Mirror*. One had read *Journal of Advanced Nursing*, one *Lancet* and *BMJ*. One said she had read some RCN monographs but could not name or describe any.

Research in nursing was considered very much less important at the time when most of these ward sisters were undertaking training for registration, but some only qualified in the late 1970s and yet not one was introduced to research during training. There was obviously no deliberate endeavour in any respect towards equipping people with an appreciation of research in nursing practice.

Before undertaking the research it seemed to the writer that there was a growing recognition among nurses that research *ought* to be increased and that findings should be used in practice. However, there did appear to be a lack of motivation about doing so and confusion about whose responsibility it was to take action to ensure that aspects of nursing care were based on those research findings that are available. The remaining questions that are included here enquire into these matters.

Q35. What do you consider to be the extent of your responsibility and the nature of your role in introducing nursing practice research findings into nursing practice?

This question was made open-ended to allow freedom of response. When necessary ward sisters were asked to say whether it was 'heavy', 'moderate', or 'slight'? The reason for asking about the 'nature of your role' was to ascertain whether they believed they should be 'active' or 'passive'. The researcher asked them to elaborate the answers given to avoid asking whether they thought they should be active or passive outright, but a small minority were asked outright − both of the alternative answers were given.

Extent of Responsibility

	Heavy	Moderate	Slight	None
Teaching (n = 12)	2	5	4	1
Non-teaching (n = 16)	5	7	3	1

Nature of Role

Teaching	Active		Passive	
	8		4	

Leader	Facilitator/ Catalyst	Informer	Follower	Allow others to do what they want	None
3	3	2	2	1	1

Non-teaching:	Active		Passive	
	11		5	

Leader	Facilitator/ Catalyst	Informer	Follower	Allow others to do what they want	None
6	2	3	2	2	1

Comment: It is clear that this is a normative question, it makes respondents answer with what they think they *should* do and not what they actually do.

Those respondents who said that they had a heavy responsibility followed this up by saying that they should take the lead.

Q36. In your ward is any particular aspect of nursing practice based on, or closely in line with, any nursing practice research findings that you have read?

The researcher explained that in order to answer yes, respondents must, on the one hand, have read a nursing practice research report, and on the other, know that actual practice is consistent with the findings.

Ward Sisters

Teaching		Non-teaching	
Yes	No	Yes	No
2	10	2	14

Q40. How important do you think it is to conduct further research into nursing practice?

	Very Important	Quite Important	Not very Important	Not Important at all
Teaching District	7 (59%)	4 (33%)	1 (8%)	0
Non-teaching District	11 (69%)	4 (25%)	1 (8%)	0

Q41. Rank, in order of importance, what you think are the reasons why more nursing practice research should be carried out

The four reasons were included in the schedule. The researcher believes them to be the four most important reasons for carrying out nursing practice research. Respondents were handed the schedule and asked to rank them, taking as much time as they felt they needed. The results are contained in Table 8.3.

Table 8.3: Ward sisters responses for reasons why more nursing practice research is required

Order of importance		Number of times ranked				Points Score* (x)	Average Individual weighting x/n
		1st	2nd	3rd	4th		
Teaching (n = 12)							
1st	To improve quality of care	12	0	0	0	48	4.0
2nd	To shorten patients' stay	0	5	4	3	26	2.1
3rd	To economise on resources	0	4	3	5	23	1.9
3rd	To enhance professionalism in nursing	0	3	5	4	23	1.9
Non-teaching District (n = 16)							
1st	To improve quality of care	13	3	0	0	61	3.8
2nd	To shorten patients' stay	1	5	7	3	36	2.25
3rd	To enhance professionalism in nursing	2	5	3	6	35	2.2
4th	To economise on resources	0	3	6	7	28	1.75

* 4 points were awarded to each first ranked choice, 3 to each second, 2 to each third and 1 to each fourth ranked choice

Note: The 'average individual weighting' is used so that a direct comparison of responses to this question can be made between any two sub-groups within the total population. The total points (x) for each 'reason' is divided by the sub-group population (n).

Thus x/n is an equated weighting factor which can be used to compare the sub-groups.

Comment. There is clearly no doubt about the strong positive orientation toward patients' welfare as evidenced by the order of importance of reasons for carrying out further nursing practice research. Comparatively little regard is paid to economy of resources as a reason for more research. This may be seen as surprising at a time of severe economic stringency and may be viewed as disappointing by those whose interest is focused on efficiency and cost effectiveness within the health service. It should be remembered that ward sisters are not budget holders and they tend to be protected from direct responsibility of financial management. Some readers may be disappointed to see what appears to be only moderate overt attention being given to the 'enhancement of professionalism in nursing'. Considering the choice of 'reasons' this is not surprising and the results speak volumes for the conception of one of the foremost ideals of professionalism, that is 'service to one's client'. The answers confirm this as the prime consideration. Unfortunately, the adoption of innovations in nursing practice, revealed by research to be of definite benefit to patients, is the exception rather than the rule. This fact negates implied notions of professionalism. In the non-teaching district the six ward sisters on geriatrics put, 'to enhance professionalism in nursing' above 'to shorten patients' stay'. This is probably because their wards have medium- and long-stay patients and it might be thought that little of practical use could be done to bring benefits to this group of patients. Another factor might be a stronger feeling than ward sisters on other wards that they need a lift in status.

Q4(a). How far do you think it is part of your role to encourage research into nursing practice?

	Very Important	Quite Important	Not an Important Part	Not Part of role
Teaching	2	6	1	3
Non-teaching	1	7	1	7

Note: It was generally found that ward sisters in both districts interpreted this question as normative. They felt it should be a part of their role, but as things were at present they could do little.

Q45. Have you read, or heard of, the following nursing practice research reports?

	Teaching (n = 12)		Non-teaching (n = 16)	
	Read	Heard of but not read	Read	Heard of but not read
(a) *Information: A Prescription Against Pain* (Hayward, 1975)	2	3	0	1
(b) *Food for Thought* (Jones, 1975)	0	4	0	3
(c) 'Pressure Area Care', Doreen Norton (in *An Investigation of Geriatric Nursing Problems in Hospital* (Norton, McLaren and Exton-Smith, 1962 and 1975)	3	4	2	4

In the teaching district the two ward sisters who said they had read (a), had read 'parts of it but not all of it', and both said it was a long time ago. When asked of the source of the copies, one said 'another hospital while on a JBCNS Course', the other could not remember. Of the three who said they had read (c), one 'borrowed the copy from a colleague about three years ago', another read it, 'years ago' but could not remember the source, the third had 'read extracts in the nursing press'.

In the non-teaching district the two ward sisters who had read (c) were asked to name the source of the copy. One had read it at another hospital while on a short course, the other had read it 'ages ago' and could not remember the source.

Only four of the twenty-eight ward sisters (14 per cent) have introduced just one innovation each, but only one actually read about the research herself, and this a brief report in a popular nursing journal. This indicates a negative attitude of nurses toward change of practice. An optimistic finding is the ranking of perceived benefits, but it must be realised that no strength of motivation can be inferred.

General Comment on Ward Sisters' Responses

The comparisons between the responses of the ward sisters from the different districts have revealed marked similarities in most cases. In the minority of instances where differences were apparent comment was made following the particular response. A disappointing feature was an obvious and generalised lack of initiative towards innovation in nursing practice as a means of improving the quality of patient care. Ward sisters were aware of what should be done in this respect but it was not translated into action. One of the main reasons for this probably lies in the almost non-stop high pressure that ward sisters have to contend with. This was obtrusively apparent through most of the interviews. It is, of course, a very well-known phenomenon of the ward sister role.

Nurse Managers

A total of fourteen nurse managers were interviewed. In the teaching district these were one divisional nursing officer, one senior nursing officer, and three nursing officers. Their age range was 36-54 years, with an average of 41.4 years. In the non-teaching district those interviewed were two divisional nursing officers, one senior nursing officer and six nursing officers. Their ages were 28-58 years, with an average of 49.3 years (one nursing officer declined to give her age).

The same questions were put to the nursing service managers as were put to the ward sisters (see Table 8.2), along with some additional questions relevant to nursing service managers. Their responses are shown in Table 8.4.

Q13. Do you keep up with nursing practice research?

Teaching		Non-teaching	
Yes	No	Yes	No
4	1	4	5

The responses to the questions in Table 8.4 show that the nursing service managers have had little opportunity made available to them for gaining an appreciation about research, but they have not taken a lead in creating opportunities for themselves or, more importantly, for the clinical nurses whom they manage. The prevailing attitude is further illustrated in response to Question 27 (a follow-up to Question 26). All four requests to nurse managers in the teaching district were from 'outside' agencies (universities). The one nurse manager (nursing officer) in the non-teaching district had been asked for help by two of her ward sisters; she had 'provided them with literature, but nothing came of it'.

The responses of the nurse managers about the responsibilities and nature of their role in the introduction of nursing practice based on research are displayed in Table 8.5.

Table 8.4: Questions to nursing service managers

		Yes	No
Q10	During your training, did you have sessions on research appreciation?	0	14
Q11	During your training, did you read nursing practice research reports?	0	14
Q12	During your training, was nursing practice taught based on particular nursing practice research reports?	0	14
Q15	Since qualifying, have you attended nursing research appreciation sessions?		
	(teaching)	4	1
	(non-teaching)	1	8
*Q17	Have you organised/run nursing research appreciation sessions?	0	14
Q20	Have you had any inservice training concerned with evaluating nursing practice research?	0	14
*Q21	Have you organised/run any such sessions	0	14
*Q23	Have you offered help to clinical staff to evaluate nursing practice research reports?	0	14
Q24	Have you requested help to evaluate nursing practice research reports?	1	13
*Q26	Has anyone requested your help on any aspect of nursing research?		
	(teaching)	4	1
	(non-teaching)	1	8
Q28	Are you aware of Nursing Research Interest Groups?		
	(teaching)	5	0
	(non-teaching)	6	3
Q29	Are you a member?	0	14
Q30	Has anyone encouraged you to attend Nursing Research Interest Groups?	1	13
*Q31	Have you publicised Nursing Research Interest Groups?	0	14
*Q32	Have you encouraged any particular person to attend a Nursing Research Interest Group?	2	12

*questions not put to ward sisters

Q14. In the teaching district three answering 'Yes' have read RCN monographs. The other had sent for and read about nursing process. Four read *Nursing Times, Nursing Mirror* and *Nursing Focus* regularly. Divisional nursing officer reads *Health and Social Services Journal.* The manager answering 'No' did not read journals regularly.

In the non-teaching district none have read RCN monographs. Eight of the managers read *Nursing Times, Nursing Mirror* and *Nursing Focus* regularly. One also read *Health Visitor and Community Nursing*. One read no journals on a regular basis. There appeared to be no difference in the reading undertaken or in any other answer given between those answering 'Yes' or 'No' to Q13.

Q35. What do you consider to be the extent of your responsibility and nature of your role in introducing nursing practice research findings? (See Table 8.5).

Table 8.5: Responses of nursing service managers about responsibility and role in the introduction of nursing practice research findings

Active/Passive Role			Both Districts		
		Div No	SNO	NO	TOTALS
A	Guiding implementation	1	1	2	4
A	Facilitating change	2	2		4
A	Encourage ward sisters to implement			3	3
P	Providing information	1		2	3
P	Familiarise myself with innovations			2	2
P	Evaluate worth of innovations	2			2
P	Monitoring that innovations were being implemented			2	2
A	Plan programme of implementation	1			1
A	*Implementation of district policy			1	1
A	'Take the lead'			1	1
P	Providing training	1			1
P	'To pass it down the line'			1	1

*active only if district policy is to implement changes

There did not appear to be any purpose in separating responses from the districts, as no differences were apparent. Respondents gave between one and four roles. The active/passive role is taken in the managerial sense, in that to be considered 'active', the role must result in action from a subordinate – in this case a ward sister.

So far it is apparent that nursing service managers have had little involvement with nursing research or its appreciation, yet they have identified what they should do to encourage uptake of findings. Two questions were asked about whether further research should be undertaken and why. Ten managers said it was 'very important' for further research to be carried out. Their reasons for saying so are given in Table 8.6.

Q41. Rank, in order of importance, what you think are the reasons why more nursing practice research should be carried out

(See Table 8.6).

Table 8.6: Nursing service managers responses as to why more nursing practice research is required

Order of Importance	Number of Times Ranked				Points Score* (x)	Average Individual Weighting x/n
	1st	2nd	3rd	4th		
Teaching (n = 5)						
1st To improve quality of care	4	1			19	3.8
2nd To enhance professionalism in nursing	1	3			13	2.6
3rd To economise on resources		1	3	1	10	2.0
4th To shorten patients' stay			2	3	7	1.4
Non-teaching District (n = 9)						
1st To improve quality of care	8	1			35	3.9
2nd To enhance professionalism in nursing	1	2	5	1	21	2.3
3rd To shorten patients' stay		4	3	2	20	2.2
4th To economise on resources		2	1	6	14	1.5

Nurse managers from both districts give maximum points, bar one, to 'improve quality of care' – showing the same strength of support for this as ward sisters. Both sets of nurse managers rank to 'enhance professionalism in nursing' second (average individual weighting – teaching 2.6, non-teaching 2.3). Both sets of ward sisters placed it third (average individual weighting – teaching 1.9, non-teaching 2.2). Nurse managers appear to place greater importance on professionalisation than ward sisters. Both groups rank highly on professional ideals, i.e. putting service to patients clearly first. However, if quality of care is enhanced by adopting innovations arising from research, and these are not adopted (which they are not), it can be argued that both groups score low on professionalism.

Nurse managers were asked, 'How far do you think it is part of your role to encourage research into nursing practice?' Nurse managers in the teaching district treated this as a normative question; four acknowledged it as part of their role, but one denied it. In the non-teaching district four of them were sure that the encouragement of research into nursing practice had nothing to do with them. They were asked to say what their role was and responded as follows:

	Encouragement of subordinates	Provision of facilities	Provision of information	Talent spotting
Teaching (n = 4)	1	2	2	1
Non-teaching (n = 5)	4	1	1	

	Identifying problems	Initiate
Teaching (n = 4)	1	
Non-teaching (n = 5)		1

In the answers given *per se* and by way of elaborating to explain what they saw as their position, it is obvious that they believe their role is encouraging further research to be passive. Only one nurse manager (of five) in the teaching district thought it part of her role to encourage subordinates to carry out research into nursing practice, against four out of nine in the non-teaching district. From the discussion around this question the researcher had the impression that research requirements were not understood.

Q45. Have you read, or heard of, the following nursing practice research reports?

	Teaching (n = 5)		Non-teaching (n = 9)	
	Read	Heard of but not read	Read	Heard of but not read
(a) *Information — A Prescription Against Pain* (Hayward, 1975)	2	3	0	2
(b) *Food for Thought* (Jones, 1975)	2	1	2	1
(c) 'Pressure Area Care', Doreen Norton (in *An Investigation of Geriatric Nursing Problems in Hospital* (1962, 1975)	4	1	3	3

Those who had read the research reports were asked to name the source of the copy.

The answers given were:

(a)   *Information – A Prescription Against Pain*
Own copy (seen by researcher in office) (1); lent by Consultant Surgeon (1).

(b)   *Food for Thought*
Royal College of Nursing Library (2) (1 teaching, 1 non-teaching); School of Nursing Library (not present district) (1) (teaching); Polytechnic Library (1) (teaching); Leverhume Foundation (1) (non-teaching); Cannot remember (2) (1 teaching, 1 non-teaching).

It will be noted that not one nurse manager borrowed a School of Nursing copy of any of these research reports from their present district, although both libraries had copies of them, and other research reports, in the main School of Nursing Library.

Overall Comment About the Responses of Nurse Managers

Comments have been made where the researcher thought it pertinent following the data to each question. It is obvious that nurse managers' perceptions and attitudes about research and their relative lack of action concerning the implementation of nursing practice innovations are serious in their implications.

In a few nurse managers, the responses made to the questions and in comments made afterwards, the main problem is role confusion. That is they were aware that there was a need for such a role to be played, but did not play that role. For the majority it was apparent that they did not even recognise that there was a need for such a role. Several openly said that only during the interview did they realise what needs to be done in this area. The researcher was aware that there was a general apprehension among the nurse managers about research. For them it was a 'beyond' area, shrouded in mysticism.

Nurse Educationalists

Nurse educationalists interviewed (both districts combined): one director of nurse education, three senior tutors, three nurse tutors, one clinical teacher. Their age range was 34-58 years with the average age of 43.8 years.

All claimed to keep up with current nursing practice research.

All read *Nursing Times* and/or *Nursing Mirror*, four read *Journal of*

Advanced Nursing, two read RCN monographs, two read other specialist learned journals.

Half of them had attended nursing research appreciation sessions since qualifying. Three from the teaching district and one from the non-teaching district had heard of Nursing Research Interest Groups, but none had attended a meeting.

The position of the nurse educationalist was in many respects at a distance from clinical nursing, but they do acknowledge that they have a direct or an indirect responsibility for clinical practice (see Table 8.7).

Q35. What do you consider to be the extent of your role and responsibility in introducing nursing practice research findings?

Table 8.7: Responses of nurse educationalists about responsibility and role in the introduction of nursing practice research findings

		Respondents		
	Director of Nurse Education	Senior Tutors	Nurse Tutors	Clinical Teacher
Passive/ Active				
P Provide information		1	2	
A Encourage subordinate teaching staff to inform and support clinical staff	1			
A Encourage ward sister to implement		3	1	
P Provide support for clinical nurses		1	1	
A Introduce research methods and findings to learners			1	
Not part of role				1

There is a close agreement between senior tutors and nurse tutors on their perceived roles. The director of nurse education did not spell out individual functions, but most could be fitted into his 'blanket' statement. It is conspicuous that no-one specifically mentioned inservice education or training for qualified staff. The impression that the researcher gained about the clinical teacher was that she 'taught what she was told to teach'.

All nurse educationalists stated that it was 'very important' or 'quite important' for further nursing practice research to be undertaken, as shown by their answers to the next question (Table 8.8).

Q41. Rank, in order of importance, what you think are the reasons why more nursing practice research should be carried out

Table 8.8: Nurse educationalists' responses as to why more nursing practice research is required

Order of Importance	Number of Times Ranked				Points Score* (x)	Average Individual Weighting x/n
	1st	2nd	3rd	4th		
Teaching District (n = 4)						
1st To improve quality of care	3	1	0	0	15	3.75
2nd To shorten patients' stay	1	2	1	0	12	3.0
3rd To enhance professionalism in nursing	0	1	1	2	7	1.75
4th To economise on resources	0	0	2	2	6	1.5
Non-teaching District (n = 4)						
1st To improve quality of care	2	1	1	0	13	3.25
2nd To economise on resources	1	1	1	1	10	2.5
3rd To shorten patients' stay	1	1	0	2	9	2.25
4th To enhance professionalism in nursing	0	1	2	1	8	2.0

In common with ward sisters and nurse managers, nurse educationalists in both districts put 'to improve quality of care' foremost. Discrimination between the four reasons is markedly stronger in the teaching district, the non-teaching district scatter being smaller.

All except one nurse educationalist (a clinical teacher) said it was important to encourage research into nursing practice. Only one mentioned a training role and one other would want to be directly involved in the research within the clinical setting.

Q45. Have you read, or heard of, the following nursing practice research reports?

	Teaching (n = 4)		Non-teaching (n = 4)	
	Read	Heard of but not read	Read	Heard of but not read
(a) *Information — A Prescription Against Pain* (Hayward, 1975)	0	4	0	3
(b) *Food for Thought* (Jones, 1975)	1	1	1	1
(c) *Pressure Area Care* (Norton, 1962 and 1975)	3	1	3	0

In the teaching district, of the four reported readings of the research reports, two of those reading *Pressure Area Care* read a copy from the School of Nursing Library, the third was unable to recall the source of the copy. The senior tutor who had read *Food for Thought* read a copy in the School of Nursing Library.

In the non-teaching district none of the three nurse educationalists, who between them declared four readings, could remember the sources of the copies.

Twenty-four readings of these nursing practice research reports are possible by the eight nurse educationaliists. Only eight readings (33 per cent) have occurred, six of these (25 per cent) about pressure area care — the only one of the three whose findings were found to have made any impact. But it must be said that no direct evidence was revealed to suggest that these readings were instrumental in this.

The most disturbing aspect is that seven of the eight had heard of Hayward's research, yet not one had read it.

Overall Comment about the Responses of Nurse Educationalists

It must be remembered that only eight were in the population but it can be assumed that nurse educationalists are a more homogeneous group than both the ward sisters and the nurse managers. Academically they are the highest qualified and, it must be said, should have fewer difficulties in gaining access to the research reports (copies of the three cited and others are available in both School of Nursing Libraries) and of understanding them. However, they need sessions on research appreciation. The School of Nursing in the teaching district is well staffed, but in the non-teaching district the School is badly under-staffed. There is controversy nationally about how much the teaching staff employed to teach learners should also teach trained staff. The source of funding for salaries is separate and is 'regionally' funded for teaching staff for nurse learners but 'district' funded for 'post-basic' educationalists. In most Schools of Nursing there is probably only a small amount of teaching of trained staff by those nurse teachers funded for basic courses. Both districts have one post-basic nurse educationalist, but neither of these were interviewed.

Although this issue can be allowed to restrict communication and cause demarcation, there was no evidence revealed to suggest that it was seen as an overt major impediment. It is more likely the case that lack of awareness and lack of commitment is because of the absence of policy about implementation of nursing practice innovations and the importance of this to the achievement of the ultimate good of higher quality patient care.

Summary of Findings from Responses to the Main Interview Schedule

There are far more similarities between the two districts than there are differences. Only two wards in each district have consciously adopted innovations known to have arisen from research. In neither district has there been any education or training specifically concerned with enabling nurses to evaluate nursing practice research findings. There is an absence of policy concerning the whole of this subject area. The little initiative that has been shown has been individually generated by a few ward sisters who have had only minimal support from nurse managers and educationalists.

In both districts there was a strong suggestion that a panel, or panels, should be set up in order to evaluate nursing practice research reports and to make recommendations concerning the adoption of innovations in nursing practice which arise from them. In both districts a minority of respondents suggested the establishment of a special post for the implementation of nursing practice innovations. Although only a few respondents advanced this idea, it was spontaneous. Had a proposal been put on this it is probable that it would have gained wider support. Lack of role clarity was widespread in all groups in both districts concerning the whole area of nursing practice research and its implementation. The widest range of perceptions was found about this with a strong tendency to believe that the role and responsibility should belong with someone else. It is clear that the issue had not been properly discussed, if at all, in either district.

A large majority of the respondents consider that there are serious impediments standing in the way of adopting innovations. Among the ward sisters who stated impediments were the only four who said that they had adopted innovations. Their responses were virtually the same as the non-adopters. This suggests that if the will is there, a way will be found.

Only 2 out of the 50 respondents, one ward sister in each district, said that it was 'not very important' to conduct further research into nursing practice. Of the other 48, 33 said it was 'very important' and fifteen 'quite important'. Some may have given what they anticipated to be the 'right' answer, but it is unlikely that there were sufficient doing so to reverse the result. All groups ranked 'to improve quality of care', the most important reason for carrying out more nursing practice research. There is clearly a difference in what nurses believe should be done to improve the quality of patient care and their actual behaviour. They make almost no effort to find out about research already done and fail to apply it when it is known.

Conclusions from the Survey

Where relevant, comments have been made under the data displayed separately for the ward sisters, the nurse managers and the nurse educationalists. Stated briefly there are marked similarities and few appreciable differences between the different grades of staff and between the districts. The differences are of degree rather than kind and indicate that the problems revealed are common to both districts. The findings are related to the hypotheses as follows:

Hypothesis A

Inservice and other post-registration training will be found to be absent or inadequate in preparing nurses to evaluate and implement findings of nursing practice research reports.

Findings. It was discovered that no nurse during her SRN course had received any tuition concerning research appreciation or read nursing practice research reports, and that no nursing practice that was taught was based on nursing practice research (Q10, 11, 12). This is not surprising in view of the comparative recency of nursing practice research.

The answer to Q15 (Since qualifying have you attended nursing research appreciation sessions?), revealed the following:

	Yes	No
Ward Sisters	0	28
Nurse Managers	6	8
Nurse Educationalists	4	4
Total	10 (20%)	40 (80%)

Not one nurse had received inservice training concerned with evaluating nursing practice research, nor had any been offered help to evaluate nursing practice research reports.

Conclusion. The findings strongly support hypothesis A.

Hypothesis B

A general lack of awareness will be found among clinical nurses and nurse managers about nursing practice innovations available in published research reports.

Findings. In addition to all nurses answering Q11 and Q12 in the negative, the responses to Q45 were predominantly negative.

There were 20 readings of the research reports by 28 ward sisters and 14 nurse managers. The total possible readings is 126. The total readings made represents 16 per cent of those possible. The number of nurses in the 'have read' plus those in the 'have heard of' category is only 40 per cent. The communication deficit is thus 60 per cent.

Conclusion. These findings give strong support to hypothesis B (as a comparison nurse educationalists have a 33 per cent reading rate and a combined reading and 'heard of' rate of 75 per cent).

Hypothesis C

Nurses do not actively seek out nursing practice research reports and read them.

Findings. Only 16 per cent of possible readings of the three cited in this research were made, the difference between having been heard of and of being read was 24 per cent; the remaining 60 per cent is a communication deficit (unawareness of the Report's existence).

Conclusion. These findings strongly support hypothesis C.

Hypothesis D

Few wards will be found to have adopted the findings of nursing practice research reports.

Findings. Only two ward sisters (in the non-teaching district), said that they had implemented Norton's findings and suggestions on pressure area care. Even this was not fully corroborated by the responses to the supplementary questions. These revealed no real difference between their practice and that of ward sisters who answered 'No' to Q36. Only two other ward sisters (in the teaching district), said that an aspect of nursing practice was in line with any nursing research findings that they had read.

Conclusion. These findings strongly support hypothesis D.

This study has been concerned with determining nurses' attitudes toward the performance of practical nursing. It has identified what ward sisters, nurse managers and nurse educationalists have or have not done to update themselves and those for whom they carry some responsibility, i.e. trained subordinates, nurse learners and nursing auxiliaries. No actual measurement of quality of patient care was attempted and no judgements about quality of patient care can be made of a quantifiable nature as a result of this investigation. What can be assumed however, is that the quality of nursing practice will be raised by basing nursing practice on objectively verified evidence revealed by rigorous scientific research.

It is undesirable for one group (say the learners) to be introduced to nursing practice innovations and not the other group (qualified nurses). This would cause great conflict and would be counterproductive. The introduction of innovation should be co-ordinated to occur simultaneously. This requires the co-operation of clinical nurses, nurse managers and nurse educationalists and the formulation of an integral local policy.

References

Briggs Report (1972) *Report of the Committee on Nursing*, HMSO, London

Brotherston, J.F.H. (1960) 'Research mindedness and the health professions' in *Learning to Investigate Nursing Problems*, International Council of Nurses and Florence Nightingale International Foundation, Geneva

Hayward, J. (1975) *Information – a Prescription against Pain*, Royal College of Nursing, London

Norton, D., McLaren, R. and Exton-Smith, A.N. (1975) *An Investigation of Geriatric Nursing Problems in Hospital*, Churchill Livingstone, Edinburgh

Report of the Royal Commission on the National Health Service (1979), HMSO, London

Wells, J.C.A. (1980) 'Nursing, a profession that dislikes innovation: an investigation of the reasons why,' M.A. Thesis, Brunel University

9 RESEARCH IN NURSING: SCHOOL OF NURSING LIBRARIES AS INFORMATION RESOURCES FOR NURSE EDUCATION

Ena Chakrabarty

I do not pretend to teach her how, I ask her to teach herself and for this purpose I venture to give her some hints . . .

Florence Nightingale

The scope and concepts in nursing have expanded considerably in the recent years. Present day nursing

involves a total specific and individual responsibility towards the patient/client and family which covers the provision of nursing, the promotion of health including health education, the prevention of illness, the indentification – by observation and reporting, of the needs of the individuals and groups and the provisions of measures to assist – both with physical, psychological, social and ethical aspects in a hospital and in the wider sector.

Moreover, nursing includes the evaluation of the care given by the nurse, the training and education of the student nurses and auxiliary staff and ability to guide other health personnel and to promote and maintain the necessary teamwork with health care staff. The nurse contributes to basic and applied research in nursing, and utilises research findings and scientific techniques resulting from continuing developments in human sciences. (Commission of the European Communities)

Education and health care are both rooted to social history and greatly dependent on current scientific and social knowledge. The philosophy and delivery of health care education is changing fast with time. The concept of acquisition of facts is being replaced with the ability to find and synthesise information and use it for problem solving. In nursing the teaching of problem solving is becoming a primary educational objective. Furthermore, 'The education of nurses and midwives is a continuous process . . . knowledge and social context is changing and new experience can and must be acquired beyond registration . . .

170

The objective of education is to improve the quality of patient care'
(Committee on Nursing, 1972). Back in 1975, the Merrison report
(DHSS, 1975) emphasised the need for the newly qualified doctor to
'recognise the limitations of his knowledge and abilities and . . . be pre-
pared for a career in medicine that is based upon continuing education'.
What is continuing education?

Continuing education should mean continuing self-education, not
continuing instruction. If this desirable goal is to be accomplished
there must be movement away from content model which encoura-
ges dependence upon teachers to a process model which demands a
significant measure of self-reliance — a shift away from preoccupa-
tion with courses and methods towards an augmented concern for
educational diagnosis and individualised therapy' (Miller, 1967).

It is this continuing education so essential to the nursing profession
that brings out the greater needs of up-to-date and reliable information
resources to back up the total education process of the profession. But
the provision of resources only is not enough — hand in hand there
should be positive efforts by all concerned with nurse education to
encourage an attitude development towards professionalism. A study
by Lamond (1974) revealed that 92 per cent of the respondents
believed that the student nurses fail to grasp that education in nursing
is a lifelong process, being part of an individual's professional responsibility which starts and does *not* finish on qualifying.

Motivated by the recommendations made in the report of the
Committee on Nursing (1972) a research project was conducted in
1977/78 in the N.W. Thames region to assess the library and information provision for nurses (Chakrabarty, 1978). This chapter is based on
some of the findings of this research, a proposed development plan that
was prepared to overcome the deficient areas and actual developments
that are taking place.

The research looked into the following areas:

(1) Library provision for the trainee and trained nursing staff in terms
of places where service points exist in the area covered by the N.W.
Thames region and access to local health care libraries.

(2) The physical environment of the library and library opening hours.

(3) Book, periodical and non-book holdings of the libraries, replace-
ment of stock and withdrawal policies; catalogues as retrieval tools.

(4)　The extent of other activities and services with special reference to communication with the user.

(5)　The extent to which these libraries were professionally staffed, and how these professionals were being utilised.

(6)　What financial resources were allocated, by whom and how they were utilised/distributed.

Two schools did not wish to take part in this survey, therefore all findings are based on 12 schools and their related districts. The survey confirmed that adequate library and information services as part of the environment necessary for professional development was very much lacking for the trained staff working in hospitals and in the community. In comparison, the library facilities for the nurses in training were found to be far better. However, in certain instances even these nursing school libraries fell far short of a desirable standard in relation to stock, services and expert/adequate staffing. Although they were all serving the training needs of nurses, having no standard guidelines, the libraries had developed independently over the years and the great disparity in provision was noteworthy.

Library Provision 1977/78

Throughout the N.W. Thames region there were 5965 nurses in training, 12 599 qualified nurses and 4078 nursing auxiliaries working in hospitals and in the community. For administrative purposes the region was divided into seven areas. These were further divided making a total of 17 districts. There were 14 Schools of Nursing to meet the basic and, in some cases, post-basic educational needs of the nurses. The schools between them provided 36 library service points.

One school had three qualified librarians responsible for each of the three site libraries, two schools had one qualified librarian each, the rest were managed by clerk-librarians. In some schools education was carried out from one main building, whereas others were multi-sited (a maximum of 5 different sites). Appreciating the fact that nursing libraries cannot provide all that may be needed by the nurses, and other libraries are of considerable help, the awareness of and accessibility to the local medical libraries were investigated. It was found that 91.6 per cent were aware of the existence of a medical library within the district. Accessibility for nurses to a medical library with or without restriction is given in Table 9.1.

Table 9.1: Availability of medical libraries to the nursing staff

Categories of Nurse	No Access	Libraries Providing		
		Reference Only	No Restriction	Access Not Known
Learners	4 (33.3%)	5 (41.6%)	1 (8.3%)	2 (16.6%)
Teaching Staff	1 (8.3%)	4 (33.3%)	5 (41.6%)	2 (16.6%)
Trained Staff in Hospital Community policies not known	2 (16.6%)	3 (25%)	5 (41.6%)	2 (16.6%)

Seventy-five per cent of the respondents felt that the medical libraries had a wealth of clinical medical information, but not necessarily geared to the nursing needs; they also felt that present day wider subject coverage needed by the nursing profession could not be sufficiently met by most of the medical libraries. Therefore, in their opinion, even though the access was there, the stock would only attract a limited number of nurses.

Access to a nursing school library for trained hospital and community nurses was found to be limited too (see Table 9.2).

Table 9.2: Access to nursing school library

Category of Nurse	Full Provision	Courtesy Provision	
		Reference	Lending
Nurses in Training	12 (100%)	—	—
Trained Nurses in Hospital	2 (16.6%)	1 (8.3%)	—
Trained Nurses in the Community	1 (8.3%)	—	—

It was agreed by the Directors of Nurse Education and the librarians that in most cases an extension of the library facility to the trained staff, without additional budget or staff would undoubtedly put a strain on the existing resources. Unless a library was particularly well-stocked and staffed, the expected demands could deprive the learner of the resources needed in the pursuance of their study. The two schools providing full services had financial help from the district management team.

In view of nurses' 24-hour duties and consequent information needs, the hours of accessibility to the library resources were looked at. It was found that none of the nurses' libraries offered accessibility round the clock. Even the medical libraries offering 'no restriction' did not provide accessibility at all times to the nursing staff. The opening hours of the main libraries in the Schools of Nursing varied from 3.5 hours to 11.5 hours a day, most common being 8-8.5 hours a day, as found in 50 per cent of the libraries. All except 2 (16.6 per cent) libraries were closed in the evenings and none were open during weekends.

It was found that very few libraries managed to impart information to their users about the various types of library services outside the parent organisation. Table 9.3 gives a breakdown of the outside library resources brought to the attention of the users:

Table 9.3: Information given to the users regarding outside libraries

Types of Libraries	No. of Libraries offering Information	% of Libraries
Professional Libraries (RCN, RCM, HVA etc)	4	33.3
Academic Libraries (Univ., Poly.)	3	25.0
Special Libraries (Wellcome, King's Fund)	3	25.0
Public Libraries (Specialisation Schemes)	4	33.3
British Library	2	16.6
Government Libraries (DHSS, DES, DOE)	2	16.6

Books, Periodicals and Non-book Holdings of the Libraries

For various reasons total bookstock of many libraries were not accurately known; the main reason was a lack of systematic record-keeping for the collections at the site libraries and the bench collections. The accounted bookstock of individual libraries varied between 2100 and 13,000, making a regional total of 72,473. The estimated total could be as much as 100,000. General reference books were few and far between, and the stock in general did not reflect outside curriculum wider reading.

Journals as a source of information were looked at. The subscription of journal titles ranged from 10 to 50, a third of the libraries subscribed to 15-19 journals, and the average was found to be 25.4.

All libraries were subscribing to current core journals. Several libraries were also subscribing to various specialist journals. Many respondents agreed that because these specialist journals had a naturally limited readership, better use could be made of them by making them available to nurses within the region. The librarians commented that in general the indexing and abstracting journals were not used by the nurses. Daily newspapers, as an important source of current news, were taken by one library and two libraries subscribed to the weekly local papers. Books and audiovisual materials complement and support each other in their contribution to teaching/learning and research and in general are regarded as part of a unified collection by the educationalists and educational technologists. The appearance of non-book materials as relevant and valuable sources of information and stimuli together with the development of new types of curricula and teaching methods have increased the need for all educational libraries to be concerned in the development of total resources available. Nurse education always had a high priority for various non-book media as teaching aids. In the present emphasis on 'continuing education', 'self learning' and 'research-mindedness' within the profession, the absolute necessity to supplement the traditional learning media of books with audiovisual and modern technological aids cannot be over-emphasised. Keeping this in mind, incorporated library stock and services were looked at.

Audiovisual resources, in all but two cases, were not included in the library catalogue. Lists of audiovisual hardware held by the schools were incomplete, and the lists of software, where occasionally found, were also incomplete. Total resources in each school, costing a considerable sum, were only used by the teaching staff and not fully utilised as learning resources by the learners as well. Absence of any recognised policy on printed and audiovisual collections in nursing schools made both these resources underutilised. Depending on the school, the responsibility for the audiovisual stock was left with a tutor, a group of tutors, librarian, audiovisual technician or a combination of any aforementioned. During the survey only two audiovisual departments had technicians in post. The relationship between these technicians with their school librarian were quite different; one was part of the library staff, so had a closer working relation, whereas the other had a vague link of an interdepartmental nature. No effective co-ordination on acquisition, collection or dissemination of audiovisual resources was found in any school.

Catalogue as a Retrieval Tool

A good catalogue to a library is what an index is to a reference book. The catalogue provides a means of access to a collection by providing a record of the total stock held at an individual library or a collection of libraries. A well-designed catalogue is a primary tool not only for the librarians, but essential for the users in gaining maximum benefit from the stock — large or small.

As the library catalogue was the most important retrieval tool it was further explored. Except in two places, the catalogues did not contain the complete holdings of any of the nursing school libraries. They listed the books held by the main library, where they were located. Often the stock of the site libraries was not catalogued at all and in general this stock was acquired and maintained by the local teaching staff. The scattered collections of a multi-sited school had a practical disadvantage, that even when a book was in stock in one of the sites, the existence of this title was frequently unknown to the user of another site. The cataloguing standard in the libraries varied with the knowledge and preferences of the library managers, as did the classification schemes. The following data on classification (see Table 9.4) will prove that instead of following a nationally-used scheme, individuality was highly valued.

Table 9.4: Classification schemes used

Classification Scheme	Number of Libraries	% of Libraries
Modified Dewey	2	16.6
RCN	2	16.6
CRC and own schemes	8	66.6

The attitudes towards a recognised classification scheme and cataloguing pattern was found very similar to what Morris *et al.* (1972) found in secondary schools.

> Librarians . . . sometimes argue that the finding mechanism employed by large libraries is necessarily elaborate . . . or that it is too difficult for their pupils to grasp. They contend that a simple arrangement of the books under the subjects that the pupils know, with a simple list or two, are most easily constructed and quite enough for all practical purposes. The fact that secondary school pupils, whatever their limitations, are probably at the height of their power of learning new things does not seem to occur to them and they do not discover for some time that the do-it-yourself mechanism they have devised − often with some trouble − is by no means simple to apply as new subjects arise or simple subjects begin to need subdivision.

In the case of nursing libraries, it was usually the nurse tutors who devised the do-it-yourself classification schemes and were greatly opposed to any changes towards a nationally-accepted scheme.

Library Services

Services excluding library orientation and user education programmes were assessed by identifying some areas, and provision by the libraries were found to be as follows in Table 9.5.

Table 9.5: Services offered by the School of Nursing Libraries

Types of Service	Number of Libraries	Total Libraries %
Accessions List	10	83.3
Information Search	7	58.3
Circulation of Periodicals	5	41.6
Subject Bibliographies	5	41.6
Subject Display	5	41.6
Selective Dissemination of Information	4	33.5
Direct Access Via Telephone	2	16.6
Interlibrary Loans	2	16.6
Other		
Students and Staff	1	8.3
Photocopy Facilities	1	8.3
Photocopy Package	1	8.3
Study Guide	1	8.3

User Education

As non-use or minimum use of libraries and literature by the nursing profession is an accepted fact (Myco, 1980; Studdy, 1980; Birch, 1979; Barrett, 1981), the survey tried to find out if any encouraging communication in the form of publicity or user education programme existed between the library and its potential users. Many respondents mentioned the lack of resources and manpower being the cause for the lack of any further publicity.

The components of the library orientation programmes carried out by the nursing schools are listed in Table 9.6.

Table 9.6: Components of the library orientation programme

Programme Consisted of	Number of Libraries	% of Libraries
Tour of the Library	12	100.0
Introductory Talk — Services	12	100.0
Introductory Talk — Resources	1	8.3
Handout Material	5	8.3
Tape/Slide Programme	1	8.3
Library Exercise/Learning Programme	2	16.6

It was found that all schools offered library orientation in the first week of training within the framework of an induction programme connected with the employment and environment. Few schools arranged a tour of the library for the trained staff during their induction week. Keeping in mind that these potential users of the library were subjected to much new information within a very short time and are likely to forget some of the information received, enquiries were made whether any school offered any back-up literature or a top-up session at any time within next three years. The answers were 'no', except at one place where a simple handout was given and occasionally the library was able to offer top-up sessions. There was no other form of user-education programme on proper use of information anywhere within the region.

In 1978 no library was found to be contributing to instil the 'research-mindedness by making sure that every nurse and midwife can use a library adequately'. Throughout the region the directors and librarians were very keen to improve their library services. Furthermore, as for the availability of resources, it was found that the total resources available within the region were substantial. With proper co-ordination and co-operation these resources could be better utilised in the most cost-effective manner.

Proposed Plan for Development of Nursing Libraries

Modern nursing needs the support of an efficient information service based on an adequate annual budget, library accommodation and service points with easy access to qualified librarians. Provision of this service is costly and the pressures on the nurse educationalists and managers are so great that it is imperative that this increasingly essential service is planned in the most economical manner possible.

The plan (Chakrabarty, 1979), was a working plan for the development of a network serving the nurses in the region. It showed a group of interconnected, mutually communicating and co-operating nursing libraries rationalising their holdings, information services and initiatives, providing prompt access at service points to all nursing and related literature, by clearly established policies and practices. In this attempt to equalise availability and quality of library service regardless of geographical location, goodwill and close collaboration was regarded to be essential between libraries and those responsible for provision and maintenance of libraries. The identification of common goals by the Regional Nurse Training Committee and the region/area/district with their differing responsibilities was needed as a contributory factor to the success of the plan.

The Development Plan – Phase 1

The suggested plan was to be implemented in three phases, with a librarian coordinating the activities. The cumulative effect of phase 1 was to provide a greatly enhanced service in the most cost-effective way. First of all the plan would enable all library personnel, including junior qualified and unqualified staff, to benefit from the advice of a senior nursing librarian when necessary and yet each library retaining its individuality to shape its services according to local user needs. Regular meetings of librarians would encourage professional development.

Secondly, coordination of certain services and routine work such as inter-library lending and cooperative cataloguing would enable provision of prompt and enhanced library services to users of even the smallest or most geographically remote library.

A third and very important benefit achieved as a combined result of the above two would especially help the nurse education division. This new co-ordinated library service with access to professional librarians would save many hours of valuable teaching staff time that was being wasted in trying to cope with library matters.

Developments Since 1979

In an era offering a combination of information handling, communication technology, learning theories, educational design and educational technology to help nurses in their professional advancement, the findings of the survey brought the already felt inadequacies to the forefront and the resulting consciousness has accentuated developments both locally and regionally. The directors of nurse education and the RNTC agreed with the principles of cooperation and encouraged the librarians to work together, with the coordinating librarian reporting back to the directors of nurse education and the RNTC with the progress.

North West Thames Nursing Librarians' Group

The success or failure in any cooperative venture is entirely dependent on the clear understanding and wholehearted cooperation of the participants themselves. Therefore before proceeding to take any action to improve the library provision, it was felt necessary that regular meetings between librarians should be considered as a first priority. It was found in the survey that the librarians in this region had a diverse background in education, training, experience, and status. Added to this, working in isolation had a professionally dampening effect on the qualified librarians. It was therefore considered essential that they appreciate the implications and expectations of their role in the present day nurse-education environment and in that light consider the proposed ideas of cooperation. The theme of the meetings gave librarians an opportunity to express their views in order to make any action a joint venture. Regular meetings and professional discussions have made librarians professionally alert, and developed a fellow feeling and interdependency by which exchange and use of information is on the increase. Having support of other colleagues, each librarian is now able to take a more positive resource-provider role.

Co-operation Between Libraries

As a first step the librarians have established a 'periodicals cooperative' by pooling their resources of some 150 titles. A *Union List of Periodicals*, updated yearly and awaiting its third edition, is used by each librarian to facilitate circulation and to promote the use of periodicals. To keep administrative procedures at a minimum it is possible to telephone a request to the library holding the periodical and a photocopy of the requested article is provided free of charge. The total number of photocopy requests made under this agreement is not known for the Region, but records kept by the Wolfson School shows that it is on the increase. The *Union List* has made the total periodical resources known and available to all nurses working in the region. It has particularly helped the users of libraries whose periodical holdings are small or whose back numbers are limited.

A directory has been compiled providing details of stock, opening hours, staff addresses and telephone numbers of the nursing libraries within the region, in order to facilitate communication. Inter-library lending of books and reports started following the success with periodical literature lent quite freely. Appreciating that physical removal of certain items may be contrary to the local users' interest, each librarian is entitled to refuse a loan. However, in keeping with the spirit of co-operation, in such circumstances the librarian normally does make her stock available for reference purposes. Often, a user studying a particular subject in depth is given permission to have direct access to the resources of another library within the region. In the first two years of the library co-operation the users did not show much response but 1981/82 saw an increase in the direct use of information resources of another library.

Union Catalogue

It is accepted that no library can hold all documents that may be requested by its users and an awareness of stock held at the co-operating libraries can help the librarians to arrive at a more rational decision on acquisition and disposal of stock. The survey found that apart from the duplicated core nursing books, the total library resources within the region also comprised a significant number of specialist books. Having no union catalogue, these specialist books were lost to all nurses except a few, and in some instances, led to duplication of highly-specialist occasionally-used items. The development plan suggested that rationalisation of total holdings within the region and production of a union catalogue of books would encourage further flow of information and utilise the total resources in the most cost-effective manner.

Co-operative Cataloguing

The development plan also suggested co-operative cataloguing in order to eliminate duplication of efforts and furthermore to: (a) achieve a good standard of cataloguing of individual holdings; (b) automatically update or create a new union catalogue of books and other learning resources resulting in benefits listed in (c); (c) provide the users with access to and knowledge of total resources of the region; (d) publish a list of new resources in the region; (e) and last, but very important, release staff to develop or improve other functions of a library as information resource centre.

With the support of additional staff and the Wolfson School of

Nursing library as a co-ordinating centre, the work on Union Catalogue and Co-operative Cataloguing are now in progress.

Library's Information Resource and the User

The library as an information resource could only be effective if its users actively seek the information they need from their library. It is only then the silent resources become suddenly active and go through a series of information processing activities directed and designed by the user, the librarian, or both, to produce a tailor-made result to suit the user's need. As far back as 1966 the World Health Organisation Expert Committee on Nursing (WHO, 1966) recognised that nurses' effectiveness is decreased where a library with adequate nursing and related technical literature is absent. Unfortunately, non-use or minimum use of literature and libraries by nurses is a commonly held fact.

Recently Treece (1971) enlightened us with: 'If nurses do not use libraries, it is often they do not know how to, they cannot find the book they want, perhaps cannot find the fact they want in the book when they have it . . .' The only appropriate action to rectify this sad situation is proper communication with the user and a well-designed user education programme. In *Resource Based Learning* Beswick's (1977) positive comment is a very apt one in the context:

> I suspect the students who have truly grasped what an index is all about and how it can be used for information searches, and who have developed confidence in the use of indexes and other retrieval devices will transfer with relative ease to the necessarily more awkward catalogue of general adult collection and be more ready to follow up their interest in a research mode. Early confidence and sympathetic preparation is the key to so much learning.

Following the awareness created by the survey results, most libraries in the region have started, in varying degrees, to communicate with their users in more than one way. Here is the progress made by the WSN library – primarily as a direct result of the survey. The benefits derived from observations, new experiences and wider reading necessitated by the survey provided the extra stimuli.

Indirect Communication. The signposting and written guidance simply constructed and attractively presented is considered to be the first and foremost communication with the user, yet all libraries were found to be inadequately signposted. Any written guidance on how to use the library catalogue or library resources were missing everywhere.

Over the years the library's signs and directions guiding the user to the resources have considerably improved as a result of the new awareness of the user's needs. Constant improvements are being made and observation kept relating to any changes. It is regarded as of great importance that the library is made easy to use, keeping in mind the user's needs.

What's New, a monthly publication of the library, communicates to the users with the information on the new resources added to the library and this is distributed widely. Every month a number of requests are received from nurses working in different areas as a result of this list. A series of information leaflets and a guide to the library services reinforce information at a time of need. A publicity leaflet is attached periodically to the hospital newsletter to publicise the library. The library telephone number is listed in the internal telephone directory, on all library books and publications, and users are invited to communicate by telephone if they wish so.

Direct Communication. The library appreciates that during the first contact with the learner, in her first week in the school as well as the new world of nursing, any great effort to 'educate' her is wasted. Her mind is too confused with the new environment, new jargon and her sudden transformation from the role of a schoolgirl to a 'nurse'. The librarian at this stage gives a library orientation which introduces the new user to the general techniques of the library usage, services and layout of the library, different kinds of stock held at the library with particular reference to the periodical literature. Every effort is made at this stage to create an atmosphere for effective communication between the user and her librarian, and impress that the library is a friendly, helpful place. Keeping in mind that using a library is a psychomotor skill, this verbal communication is followed by a simple questionnaire, which actually involves the learner in using the library effectively.

The skills in the use of library resources should ideally be developed with increased complexity and in phases; however the nurses' education programme is tightly packed, with hardly any room for further user education. Universities and polytechnics are increasingly taking steps to ensure that the students are educated in the use of information resources. The Academic Board of Plymouth Polytechnic has placed the use of learning resource centre within the framework of course provision. Durham University students are timetabled for instruction on the scope of the library and techniques needed for using the facilities at regular intervals throughout their course. It is recognised that for creating a healthy appetite for new or modified information a nurse not only needs formal library induction, but also tuition at regular intervals to feel competent in using all types of library resources. Lamond's survey (1974) showed that large majorities (72 per cent and 70 per cent) of the respondents considered the college of nursing to be the most appropriate venue and the first year to be the ideal time to instil a very important aspect of nursing professionalism; the nurses' own responsibility is to continue her education and be up-to-date with current professional literature.

In order to make the nurses more aware of need for continuing self education and researchmindedness, the library has been organising bi-monthly study days for the trained staff with the objectives that each participant, at the end of the day, would: (a) be able to choose a library or information centre most appropriate to the information required; (b) be aware of the library and information network that exists to help anyone seeking information; (c) know various information tools, i.e. indexes, abstracts, catalogues, that could be used to locate information sources — generally and in our own library; (d) be able to compile bibliographical references on a subject of their choice, using bibliographical tools during the workshop session; and (e) be aware of the workings of the automated information sources, etc.

Between October 1980 and April 1982 eight study days were held and these were attended by the following grades of nurses (Table 9.7).

Table 9.7: Grades of staff attending the library information day

Senior Nursing Officer	9
Nursing Officer	9
Sister/Charge Nurse	32
Clinical Teacher	5
Staff Nurse	2
Health Visitor	6
District Nurse	6

The morning session contained a tour of the library, talk on information sources including books, journals, government and semi-official publications, catalogues, indexes, abstracts, computerised retrieval and library co-operation. This was followed by a discussion. The afternoon session was mainly devoted to finding information, and methods of literature search were discussed, followed by a practical session when the participants searched for information on a subject of their choice.

Originally, the idea of a study day of this kind was inspired by Senga Bond's Information Workshop as described in Chapter 10, however the main difference is that this programme is open to nurses from all specialties. Specific subjects were dealt with in the afternoon during the practical session, when the participants were given extra help and guidance in locating specialised literature related to their searches.

Initially letters were sent to Senior Nursing Officers asking for nominations, stressing that no more than ten people should attend so that proper interaction and full participation is encouraged. On receipt of the nominations, the nominees were sent a letter enclosing a programme inviting them to attend the day. A booklet describing the organisation of library resources and systematic approach to information search was also enclosed with the letter for them to read before they attended the Study Day (Chakrabarty, 1981). A questionnaire was given to each participant at the end of the day to evaluate their response. This was supplemented by discussion taking the points raised by the participants. The participants' replies to the most and least useful items of the day were as follows (Table 9.8).

Table 9.8: Most and least useful programmes

Topics Discussed/Programme Participated	Most Useful	Least Useful
Index, Abstracts, Catalogues	43	1
Government Publications	2	7
Computerised Information Sources	2	4
Literature Search — Theory and Practical	34	1
Scope of the Library: Looking Around	13	—
Outside Resources	8	—
Getting to Know the Librarian and Librarian's role	14	—

Forty-one and twenty-four participants, respectively, found the day's programme very useful and all except one found participation in the programme worthwhile. Comments like 'I now know that I *can* use the library fully, there are no "mysterious areas" to stay away from' and '. . . also knowing the librarian personally, I feel quite happy about phoning up about a query which I would not have done before', makes us feel that communication with the user is flowing in the right direction.

Often, on arrival, the participants who had not used libraries for any other purpose than borrowing books, were unsure of the content of the day, but as the aims and objectives were explained once again during the introduction, and the interactive programme of the day followed, they felt comfortable and some were even excited at being able to find information for themselves. The aim of the day was not to overload the participants with librarianship jargon, but to stress that if looked for methodically, information was easy to find, and that there was a friendly librarian around to help if needed.

Conclusion

'To gather knowledge and to find out new knowledge is the noblest occupation of the physician. To apply that knowledge . . . with sympathy born of understanding to the relief of human suffering is his loveliest occupation.' This comment made by Edward Archibald (1968), is equally applicable to present day nursing. In this era of information explosion when the seekers for new knowledge are bewildered by the vast quantity of information available and the various technological and sophisticated means of accessing them, the nurses have an added problem; the nursing in this country at present is experiencing some radical changes in its educational structure and professional attitude. Never before was the nurses' need greater for prompt availability of information and access to professional expertise in information handling. In this continuum of nurse education and professionalism the nursing school library with its powerhouse of resources is a natural place to offer nurses the backup they need by collecting, disseminating and teaching to handle relevant information. To carry out this role successfully the library must constantly research into the changing needs of its user to whom Florence Nightingale advised: 'Let us not consider ourselves as finished nurses . . . we must be learning all our lives'.

Further Reading

Atthill, C. (1978) 'The cure for decidophobia', *Times Educational Supplement*, 7 July 1978, p. 41

Binger, J.L. and Jensen, L.M. (1980) *Lippincott's Guide to Nursing Literature*, Lippincott, Philadelphia

Brake, T. (1980) *The Need to Know*: *Teaching the Importance of Information* — Final Report for the period of January 1978-March 1979, Report No. 5511, British Library Lending Division, London

Department of Education and Science (1975) *A Language of Life*: Report of a Committee of Inquiry appointed by the Secretary of State for Education and Science under the Chairmanship of Sir Alan Bullock, HMSO, London

Noble, P. (1980) *Resource Based Learning in Post-Compulsory Education*, Kogan
Page, London

References

Archibald, E. (1968) Quotation in Strauss, M.B. (ed.), *Familiar Medical Quotations*, Little, Brown and Co, Boston, p. 256

Barrett, D.E. (1981) 'Do nurses read? Nurse managers and nursing research reports,' *Nursing Times, 77*, 2131-4

Beswick, N. (1977) *Resource Based Learning*, Heinemann Educational Books Ltd, London

Birch, J. (1979) 'Nursing should be a research based profession,' *Nursing Times* Occasional Paper, *75*, 135-6

Chakrabarty, E. (1978) A Survey of Library Provision for Trainee and Trained Nurses in the N.W. Thames Region (Unpublished Report)

Chakrabarty, E. (1979) A Suggested Plan for Development of Nursing Libraries in the N.W. Thames Region (Unpublished).

Chakrabarty, E. (1981) *Looking for Information*, Wolfson School of Nursing of Westminster, London

Commission of the European Communities Advisory Committee on Nursing (1980) *A Report of the Training of Nurses Responsible for General Care, in particular on the balance to be found between Theoretical and Clinical Instructions for this Category of Nurse*, Brussells, Committee of the European Community, Doc. Ref. 111/D76/6/80 - EN

Committee on Nursing *Report* (1972) Chairman: Prof. Asa Briggs, HMSO, London

DHSS (1975) The Committee of Inquiry into the Regulation of the Medical Proffession *Report.* Chairman: Dr A.W. Merrison, HMSO, London

Lamond, N. (1974) *Becoming A Nurse*, Royal College of Nursing, London

Miller, G.E. (1967) 'Continuing education for what?' *Journal of Medical Education*, April, 1967, No. 12, 324

Morris, C.W. *et al.* (1972) *Librarians in Secondary Schools*, Schools Library Association, London

Myco, F. (1980) 'Nursing research information – are nurse educators and practitioners seeking it out?,' *Journal of Advanced Nursing, 16*, 637-46

Studdy, S. (1980) 'A computerised survey of learning needs,' *Nursing Times, 76*, 1084-7

Treece, E.W. (1971) 'The library from the nursing educator's point of view,' *Bulletin of Medical Library Association, 59*, 444-9

World Health Organisation Expert Committee on Nursing (1966) *Fifth Report*, WHO, Geneva

10 PROMOTING RESEARCH UTILISATION THROUGH INFORMATION SERVICES

Senga Bond

The preceding chapter has outlined the importance and development of library resources for nurses in one health authority from the perspective of a health service librarian. This chapter will demonstrate how a nurse, with a specific interest in the development of the conduct, utilisation, and teaching of research, has worked with libraries and librarians to facilitate greater attention to library and information services. Three developments which have taken place in the Northern Region of England since 1978 are discussed. These can be described generally as a regional library and information service for nurses, an educational programme about information called Information Workshops and a resource for nurse teachers to assist in using research findings in their teaching, called Nursing Topics.

The background to a nurse becoming so involved in information and library work stems from the unusual characteristics of my role. Briefly, this encompasses the development of all aspects of research for nurses in the Northern Region. This includes involvement in the teaching of research at all levels from basic nurse education through to the supervision of postgraduate degrees. Encouraging nurses to use research findings in their work inevitably created demands on me to produce research reports and findings relevant to nurses' problems. I found myself being contacted by procedure committees as well as individual nurses, midwives and health visitors to supply research reports on topics as diverse as nursing itself. Nurses who wish to pursue studies also require assistance to carry out literature searches as a basis for developing their project. It was obvious that for research to develop in any way then a necessary prerequisite was to have good library and information resources. Of course this in itself could not stimulate research development, but without it the chance of progress would be much reduced.

A Regional Library and Information Service

A report by the National Health Service Regional Librarians' Group (1978) showed the Northern region to be the poorest of English regions in terms of employment of professional library staff. No qualified librarians were employed in School of Nursing libraries although a few excellent multi-disciplinary libraries existed. However, in some districts, there was no library provision for qualified nurses. It was against this background that moves were made to develop a regional service rather than specific district library services. It was anticipated that interest shown for a central service would promote districts to examine their own provision. Negotiations to develop the service were protracted.

All health service personnel have access to the facilities of the University of Newcastle upon Tyne medical library. This library had decided not to develop its nursing stock in favour of Newcastle Polytechnic where a number of nursing courses had been in existence for several years. The Polytechnic was fortunate in having a Faculty Librarian who was also a nurse and who had developed an excellent nursing collection. Agreement was eventually reached with the Regional Health Authority that the Polytechnic would provide a service to nurses and paramedical staff for an initial period of two years from October 1979. A librarian was appointed with specific responsibility for the Regional Service which, from the outset, was intended to be an information rather than a library service.

To assist development of the service discussions were held with interested groups of nurses to ascertain their needs. Promotion was facilitated by the appointment of a member of staff in each district who was responsible for liaison with the Polytechnic Library. In some instances this was a member of a district library staff, but other personnel, including administrators, inservice-education officers, and nurse teachers were also appointed. The service which has evolved comprises eight main features.

Borrowing of Books and Audiovisual Stock

This may be done through an NHS librarian or directly by users telephoning or calling personally. During the first 12 months issues totalled 4816 items. Now the number of items on loan at any one time averages 1113. While the majority of loans were in health sciences and nursing almost every other subject category was borrowed. Particularly important has been the centralised audiovisual collection.

Borrowing has been facilitated by providing NHS libraries with microfiche catalogues of the book and audiovisual stock as well as journal holdings. This has the added advantage of assisting unqualified NHS library staff to catalogue their own stock.

An additional resource for borrowing has been transportation of materials to the users' district by the already existing regional van service. A recent survey by the University Medical Library (Bramley, 1982) which also relies on the regional van service, shows this to be a cheap and efficient method of distribution.

Photocopying of Stock

The requests for photocopies of articles held in the Polytechnic has shown a steady growth since the service began. Charges are made quarterly to District Health Authorities at the standard Polytechnic rate. An average of 1584 pages are being photocopied monthly compared with 181 at the beginning of the service and 666 a year after it began.

Health Information Service Bulletin

Requests for photocopies are linked with the success of a monthly current awareness service called Health Information Service (HIS). This has proven to be an excellent aid to librarians who have few bibliographical sources, as well as speeding their literature searches enormously.

Literature Searches

Providing literature searches has been an important aspect of the service. Updating of existing searches has demonstrated the value of centralised holdings of bibliographies. Inclusion of a list of completed searches in HIS has increased demand for them.

Books on Approval

The books-on-approval service was set up in conjunction with the Publishers Association to permit nurses and librarians to inspect books as a basis for purchasing decisions. Two copies of new books are received, one held permanently on display at the Polytechnic and the other for circulation to users. A list of acquisitions is circulated. To date some users have found it extremely useful, but its future is threatened by the high cost for a small number of users.

User Education

Polytechnic staff have become involved in user education in districts where there is no librarian or no librarian prepared to undertake user education. Some nurses now attend the Polytechnic library as part of their course work. Polytechnic staff also teach in NHS institutions as well as other educational establishments which run nursing courses, but which do not have specialist librarians. User education has been facilitated by the development of a Health Studies User Education package.

Ad Hoc Information

Inevitably as knowledge of the availability of the Polytechnic library service has grown so *ad hoc* requests for specific information have increased. Being able to have an instant response if at all possible has proven to be a most welcome feature of the service.

Advice to NHS Librarians

Because many workers in NHS libraries are not professional librarians they have turned to the Polytechnic staff for assistance in developing their own libraries and user education.

An evaluation of the service was carried out eighteen months after it had been set up (Bond, 1981). This showed how useful staff had found it, particularly among community staff who do not have ready access to NHS libraries. Nurse teachers also make substantial use of the service despite their being relatively well provided for in comparison with their clinical and managerial colleagues in the NHS. A review of the service resulted in the decision that the liaison scheme with districts should continue and added impetus would be given to those districts which showed least development in library use. Increased funding for the service was secured for a further three years from the Regional Health Authority and monitoring of the service will continue during this time. A centralised service like that described may not be the most suitable form for all regions, but where there is gross inequality of provision across districts and budgets have not been made available for libraries for qualified nurses, then the Polytechnic service, capitalising on already existing resources, has proven to be a highly successful and cheap option for the purposes of this region.

Information Workshops

The development of information workshops actually precedes the establishment of the library and information service. The workshops were developed while negotiations for the service were taking place during 1978 with the aim of stimulating awareness of the need for library provision and information skills among nurses.

Newcastle Polytechnic had for many years provided information retrieval courses for nurses, organised between the library and the Department of Librarianship. The experience gained through these courses provided a basis from which to develop further. A small grant from the Regional Health Authority financed production of materials and a short inservice course in information skills was produced.

Information skills is rather an abstract topic. It was conceived as having three broad components. The first was defining what kind of information is wanted – primary sources, reviews, statistics, recent or historical sources. The second aspect included how to get information from the system – general skills of information retrieval as well as knowledge of resources available locally. The third component was involved with exploiting the information retrieved, abstracting it from its source, evaluating it, synthesising and storing it. Information utilisation was regarded as the end-point of a whole series of events, whether information is acted upon, stored for further use or rejected.

In developing the course, objectives were set in seven broad areas: defining information needs; selecting publications; selecting information from documents; comparing documents; synthesising information; report writing; bibliographical references.

For the purposes of this project our target group were nurses in the ward sister and nursing officer grades whom we considered were unlikely to have had much teaching on this topic. We could have selected any grade of nurse and developed teaching material appropriate to their job. As well as concentrating on one particular grade of nurse we also planned to focus on one specialty so that there would be a common interest. (For example, we did not think that midwives would be particularly interested, professionally, in the care of the aged.) In order to select the broad subject matter for the workshops we asked area nursing officers to determine which would be most appropriate for them. They selected two sources, nurses working in psychiatry and those working with geriatric patients. Because we were constrained financially and by time to produce only one set of materials our compromise was to provide a course relevant to those working in psycho-geriatric areas.

The plan was to develop and test the materials with six groups of nurses, each group drawn from a single district or area. Applications were received by leafleting the three areas in the Northern region which had agreed to participate. In all 135 nurses were interested in participating. From this group 60 eventually took part and, because of the geographical distribution, a total of seven groups were created.

Teaching was organised to take place within the nurses' district or area within the format of workshops. All manner of group endeavours are fashionably called workshops. Our intention was that a small number of nurses should engage in a high degree of participative learning. To facilitate this exercises were developed for each section of the subject matter and these were compiled into a workbook. Participants worked through the exercises associated with each aspect of teaching at the appropriate part of the course. The subject matter was grouped into six broad topics: sources of information; comparing information and documents; extracting information from documents; preparing and writing reports; using libraries; using information in practice.

To facilitate teaching a handbook was produced containing a substantial collection of material corresponding to the six sections above. This was sent out in advance of attending the workshops and would remain the property of the participants afterwards.

In order to orientate the students to this scheme, a set of pre-workshop exercises was also developed. Some of these involved critique and interpretation of short passages and some were of a more bibliographical nature. Rather than stimulating participation, in some cases they had the opposite effect and a few nurses withdrew.

The Workshops

The total course was planned to extend over two days in any combination of whole or half days according to local convenience. In the event a variety of patterns were selected. Two or three leaders attended each workshop to contribute nursing and librarianship skills and orientations and to assist individuals to work through the exercises. A number of methods were used in the workshops, exercise completion being the main one associated with discussion of the exercises. Other methods included a tape slide, a display of publications, handling of indexes and abstracts and short (ten minute) lectures. The times allocated to different sections of the material were flexible in order to devote attention to issues raised by participants. The ordering of subject matter was also flexible to try different schemes at different workshops.

Evaluation Methods

Evaluation was both summative and formative. It was formative in the sense that we used comments made by participants in earlier workshops and acted upon these to change the presentation of later ones. Participants were encouraged to express their views at any stage of the workshop and its essentially experimental nature was stressed. Each introductory session presented opportunities for comment about the preworkshop exercises we had set and about the handbook and organisation. It was obvious that we had allowed insufficient preparation time and presented a large volume of material to nurses who were not used to this. Remarks were noted as they emerged and participants were asked to express their views on the various sections of the workshop and its relevance.

Observations of activities in the workshops included expressions of application and motivation, difficulties encountered, the nature of discussion, and all of these added texture to our assessment of work accomplished and presented in the workbooks. In addition, summative evaluation was employed using a questionnaire immediately on completion of each workshop as well as by a postal questionnaire sent out some eight months after completion to assess various aspects of behaviour related to information and reading. We found it extremely difficult to develop short tests to assess gains in the kinds of skills we were attempting to teach. It is relatively easy to test bibliographical skills by multiple choice items, but not the more complex skills of comparing and synthesising information.

Findings

Only a brief description of findings can be presented here but a full report is available elsewhere (Bond, Stephenson and Wallace, 1979). A major finding was that we had expected too much of our participants by presenting them with both subjects and methods of learning which were new to them. Many were frustrated because they could not complete their exercises and felt they had neither time to assimilate material or judge their own performance. This was despite how amazingly hard-working participants had been. More practice was required. Some nurses reported that they were grappling with too many new things at once; the setting, the workshop format, the particular exercises, the topics we were trying to introduce, and the language of the articles. In other words we had overloaded them.

Not all of the participants found the content relevant to their needs. We obtained comments like: 'We would not need to compare information. We rarely received two papers on one subject. Our policies are set', and 'Preparing detailed reports never arises in our work', 'We are not interested in figures and graphs'.

There is an obvious need to relate the materials to the clinical interests of participants. If the subject matter for example was then regarded as irrelevant, the information topic to which it was addressed was devalued. On the other hand, some found papers and extracts so interesting that they became absorbed in them and forgot about set exercises! There is obviously a need to develop appropriate materials which are short and which are also very relevant in order to sustain interest.

Of course the crux of the matter was whether the content was regarded as of value by participants and whether attendance at the workshops actually produced changes in behaviour.

Table 10.1 shows how subjects were ranked in terms of interest. The wide distribution shows no topic of supreme interest while a sizeable proportion found it difficult to say which topic was of least value. The more conceptually difficult topics, extracting and comparing information, were regarded as most difficult to understand. The results suggest however that no aspect of information use that was included in the workshop proved to be so irrelevant, or lacking in value to participants as to make it totally redundant. Therefore topics themselves were quite favourably rated.

Table 10.1: Nurses' rating of workshop topics

| | | Of Most Interest | | |
	Now	Before Workshop	Of Least Value	Most Difficult to Understand
Sources of info.	11	11	2	2
Extracting info.	17	5	5	15
Comparing info.	4	–	10	19
Report writing	15	13	5	8
Using libraries	13	8	3	4
Case study	10	16	7	–
Others				
All	1	–	–	1
None	–	1	–	1
Not sure	–	1	–	1
No response	1	6	17	9

A further 4 reported that all topics were of value

A follow-up questionnaire was sent to participants eight months after completion of the workshop. The response rate was 66 per cent, reasonable for a postal questionnaire with no reminder. We were interested in finding out whether reading habits and attempts to find information had changed, whether the report writing skills had developed, and whether the handbook retained by participants had been used at all. Participants had already given a lot of time to the workshop so the questionnaire was kept as brief as possible.

At no time had we attempted to find out how much reading associated with work the nurses actually did, but our impression was that there were few attempts to go beyond the popular nursing weeklies. In response to our question asking about amount read, just over half (57 per cent) indicated no difference in quantity while the remainder said they read more. Of course we had no way of assessing the validity of these responses. Table 10.2 shows the kind of changes brought about in terms of different kinds of publication and types of publication. Among those who report changes, the greatest change occurred in respect of new journals and items devoted to research and clinical topics. The largest number (24) reported reading more clinical material and indicated an increased volume of reading (16), suggesting an increase in this type of material read with a reduction in some other type. Changes in reading volume however are under-reported or increased interest in clinical materials are over-reported. When asked about reading skills about one-third felt they read more quickly while the remaining two-thirds said they had not changed. A small amount of practice of reading skills had been included in the workshop and while we would not have expected the speed to change, there may have been some changes in ability to locate and identify relevant points more quickly. In fact, 75 per cent said that this was the case and the remainder felt that they had not developed the skill. Equally important, 73 per cent felt that they could summarise the content of the reading better. Responses to open-ended questions suggested that participants were being more thoughtful and discriminating in what they read and how they set about reading it. Particularly evident were comments indicating an increased awareness of the need to identify main points more quickly.

Table 10.2: Nurses' reading habits

	Yes	%	No	%	Don't Know	%	No Response	%
New journals or magazines	19	51.4	14	37.8	0	0	4	10.8
Different kinds of books	8	21.6	21	56.8	0	0	8	21.6
More research type books	13	35.2	17	45.9	1	2.7	6	16.2
More clinical material	24	64.9	7	18.9	0	0	6	16.2
More difficult items	8	21.6	20	54.1	1	2.7	8	21.6

We had not asked how much effort nurses put into trying to obtain information from the many available sources, but we were interested to know whether attending the workshop had influenced their efforts. It must be borne in mind that this project took place before the establishment of the Regional Library Service. Half of our sample said they now made more frequent attempts to locate information whilst 35 per cent said they were unchanged in their behaviour and a further 10 per cent did not know. This increase was associated with greater library use for 30 nurses, though 20 reported no such increase. Of the respondents, 16 (40 per cent) had used the library for work-related purpose since the workshop. Among those who did use the library one-third said that they were able to do so much more efficiently by making better use of reference and bibliographical materials.

Of our sample, only 14 respondents indicated that they had written a report other than a kardex or staff appraisal since the workshop. This reinforces the view of many participants who did not regard report-writing as being relevant to the ward sister grade. Nevertheless, we had some responses that skills and report-writing had changed, with eleven saying that they had changed layout, thirteen had changed organisation, and twenty said they had improved their ability to summarise and express themselves.

We had allowed respondents to retain their handbooks and about one-third had used them since the completion of the workshops. This was for different reasons. Some were involved in Open University studies or Joint Board of Clinical Nursing Studies Courses and had used the handbook in assisting preparation for them. Some had used it in association with teaching of students or to help prepare comments for reports for the Nursing and Midwifery Advisory Committee. Some simply indicated that they had referred to particular sections. This suggests that those who were motivated to exercise some of the skills and ideas stimulated by the workshop found the handbooks a useful aid and some permanent record and would be a worthwhile component for courses of this kind.

At the end of the questionnaire respondents were asked whether they thought the workshop was worthwhile, not worthwhile or whether they were uncertain. None of the respondents had the courage to say that it had not been a worthwhile experience. Sixteen remained uncertain at this stage of the value of having attended. The remainder regarded attending the workshop as worthwhile. We had not obtained feedback from nineteen of our original participants. Some of the comments at the end of the questionnaires were very telling. We knew we had set out with over-ambitious goals and that we would only begin a process which is very complex. We had not set out to solve all the problems of the NHS but one comment was:

> the workshop has been very instructive but I am afraid it has not helped me very much in my job. Perhaps it has made me more aware, identify main points of articles I have read, and summarise main points more quickly, but it has not changed my job or made it any easier. I am still having to struggle to find beds for readmissions . . .

In effect, this person said we have helped them in some of the skills we set out to teach but there seems to be little value associated with these skills when struggling through the day-to-day work. This raises the issue of whether in fact there is any point in continuing with this exercise and try to teach nurses in these grades the kinds of skills which we set out to teach them.

It was evident that a number of our nurses were very interested in clinical developments and that we were right to try to slant the workshops towards a nursing specialty. However, the responses of our participants demonstrated that they did not regard seeking out new developments and adding to their own knowledge through critical reading as their responsibility. We are faced with the dilemma of whether the first step in any future development should be a stimulation of professional commitment to initiate information use or whether such workshops should be limited to those nurses who readily regard literature use as an appropriate nursing activity and show a desire to develop the skill. We may also need to consider ways of providing information to nurses which they can handle and this poses all manner of questions about current information systems. A current development stemming from these workshops is to develop the teaching of information skills to nurses attending management courses where handling information of different kinds may be regarded as more relevant to their work. Efforts are now being devoted to assess what nurse managers regard as their information needs.

Nursing Topics Project

The third development to be described is called the Nursing Topics Project. This project evolved from a recognition that nurse teachers were being asked to include research in all basic and post-basic nursing courses and that they required different kinds of assistance to do so. One means of including research in a meaningful way is to associate research projects and their findings with particular aspects of nursing being taught rather than teach research as a compartmentalised subject (Bond, 1982). In order to facilitate this, nurse teachers need to have research reports in a readily available form. Research relevant to nursing spans an enormous range of subjects and is located in an equally wide range of academic journals. Few schools of nursing in the region can boast a library with the resources to obtain this material and few tutors, even if they have the interest, have the time to engage in wide literature searching on their own behalf. The project which is described represents an attempt to capitalise on the library resources at Newcastle Polytechnic to the benefit of nurse teachers throughout the region, as well as beyond it.

The objective of the project is to produce a resource in the form of collections of selected research reports on topics relevant to nursing. Anyone who has carried out a thorough literature search knows how difficult it is to select items from bibliographical details alone. An important element of the project involves scrutinising the literature, discarding non-research or poor quality articles and retaining those that are of good quality, are relevant to nursing practice and to nurse education. To facilitate using the articles, an annotated bibliography is produced which is organised into appropriate categories within the major topic. This is aimed at facilitating selection of those articles which are appropriate to the subject being taught. To complete each unit a list of audiovisual teaching aids, any information about them and how they may be obtained is included.

The idea of producing Nursing Topics units was discussed widely with nurse teachers throughout the region. This was not only to publicise their development but to seek co-operation in their evaluation. It was also important to obtain their advice about the kinds of topics most relevant to their needs as well as the appropriate range of items to be included.

After an initial round of discussions a number of options were open about the topics regarded as most relevant and how the material should be organised. It was decided to produce units on topics offering very different scope. To date five units have been produced. These are: Mother/Infant interaction — 64 items; Temperature taking — 43 items; Reality orientation — 42 items; Management of indwelling urinary catheters — 50 items; Body image — 51 items. The numbers of research articles included in each one is shown alongside.

We began with Mother/Infant interaction. There has been an enormous outpouring of literature in recent years on this subject. It was selected however because the person with primary responsibility for developing the units is a midwife and it was thought desirable to have a first topic about which she had some knowledge, but which would generalise beyond midwifery. The remaining four topics are much narrower in scope and consequently there is far less literature available. This is reflected in the size of the units produced.

An arbitrary five years was decided as inclusion time for literature, but where research classics are involved or where findings have not been surpassed, then articles older than five years have been included.

For three of the units the literature and annotated bibliography have been assessed and amended by a nurse with specialist interest in and a knowledge of the subject. It was felt this would assist in creating a better quality product. It is gratifying that on the whole few changes have been suggested. Selection of the literature for one unit was carried out entirely by a psychologist and the remaining unit has been produced completely in house.

Because this was regarded as a pilot exercise, and in order to defray copyright costs for reproducing the articles, only ten copies of each unit have been produced on a very slim budget. We did, however, request permission from copyright holders even for this small number and obtaining their permission has added considerably to production time.

Publicity was given to the project through a short press release to the nursing newspapers and journals. This asked tutors to apply to use the units and assist in their evaluation by completing a questionnaire. Initially only three units were available but even with this very meagre publicity requests to use the units have been as follows: Mother/Infant – 101 requests; Temperature taking – 69 requests; Reality orientation – 89 requests; Management of indwelling urinary catheters – 36 requests; Body image – 40 requests.

Evaluation has been carried out by the means of a questionnaire sent with each unit. Units may be borrowed for one month. They are sent to applicants together with prepaid return postage in envopak bags. To date all units have been returned and a total of 160 completed questionnaires and 3 blank questionnaires have been received. No attempt has yet been made to analyse the completed questionnaires but data will be yielded about the organisation, content and quality of the bibliography, the literature and the section on audiovisual aids. We will also be interested to learn how and with whom the units are, or could be, used and how readily users can obtain this range of literature from other sources.

Overview

Together the library and information service, the Information Workshops, and the Nursing Topics project represent the most tangible products of a fruitful liaison between a library and department of librarianship which are wholly without the National Health Service and nurses in the sixteen districts which comprise the Northern region.

An attempt has been made to stimulate all nurses' awareness of the need to use information, not least of it research literature, and to provide the resources to satisfy that need. Whether the initiatives described will show the ultimate payoff in terms of quality of patient care depends on a complex interplay of factors. Only two of these include an awareness of new developments and the resources to ascertain whether current practices are the most efficient and effective available. If nurses are to devote their expensive time to nursing, teaching nurses or managing the service, then they have a right to supportive facilities to enable them to do so effectively. Information services are one such resource.

In this case there was no major demand from nurses in the region to improve the quality of their library information services. An absence of demand is not an equivalent to an absence of need and the takeup of the services being provided is a clear demonstration of the worthwhile quality of a small investment for an agreed trial period. Nursing could surely benefit from more trials with new low cost ideas which are carefully evaluated.

References

Bond, S. (1981) An evaluation of Newcastle Polytechnic Library Service to the Northern Regional Health Authority (unpublished)

Bond, S. (1982) 'The research component in SRN education,' *Nurse Education Today, 2,* 5-10

Bond, S., Stephenson, J. and Wallace, E. (1979) *Information Workshops for Nurses,* Report of an Evaluative Pilot Study, Newcastle upon Tyne Polytechnic

Bramley, K. (1982) Personal communication

National Health Service Regional Librarians Group (1978) Census of Staff Providing Library Services to NHS Personnel

CONCLUSION

Bryn D. Davis

The historical review in the General Introduction indicated the need for a search for increased effectiveness in the selection and recruitment of entrants to nursing. The consideration was that more suitable entrants would be more likely to become successful nurses, a somewhat circular argument. It was the hope of the profession that this would improve standards of care, as well as maintaining the service.

Developments have also occurred, organisationally, in order to improve the system: the introduction of the second portal to enrolment; the separation of nursing education from administration; the development of the study block system; changes in the syllabus.

Much of the development that has occurred over the last few years has been as a result of the Report of the Committee on Nursing and its recommendations (1972). The major development latterly has been the new legislation embodied in the Nurses' Act (1979), and the establishment of the United Kingdom Central Council and the National Boards to replace the General Nursing Councils. New syllabuses and schemes of training have been and are being developed (for example, GNC Scotland, 1978), and loosely based on the modular scheme advocated by the Committee on Nursing (1972). These aim to attain a greater integration of theory and practice within each module, with evaluation being an integral part, successful achievement of objectives being necessary before procession to the next module is allowed. Flexibility is also part of the new schemes in that a range of modules is available, depending on the resources of the particular school or college of nursing, and its associated clinical areas.

However, the system still remains one that is general, and imposed on all learners, who are selected on the basis of relatively simplistic criteria (in terms of school leaving certificates or equivalents), and then given information and experience according to the requirements of the educational body (at present the GNCs) and of the clinical areas.

A major factor in recent developments in the management of patient care has involved the use of individual care plans implemented on the basis of patient needs, problems, and clinical requirements identified from nursing assessment procedures on admission, together with the clinical medical diagnosis and prescriptions. This approach to patient care, known as the Nursing Process, has been accepted by the GNCs as the model of nursing on which nurse education and training is to be based, and with respect to which the curriculum should be developed.

The Report of the Committee on Nursing (1972) argued that nursing should become a research-based profession; research should be established as a function or role within the profession; research findings should form the basis or care strategies. As well as these developments however the Process model itself is research-based in that the nursing body of knowledge is built up from the continued monitoring of planned interventions. The recent studies of nurse education, including those in this volume, can be seen as leading to the conclusion that a similar model could usefully be applied to the education and training of nurses.

Table 1 shows the parallels between the Research Process, the Nursing Process and the Education Process. Table 2 shows in more detail the application of the model to education and training. To date the current training starts at the implementation phase, with the planning not generally being an ongoing, monitored process, related to the learners' needs. A set curriculum, developed with reference to GNC and health service requirements, and generalised stereotyped learner needs, is set up and imposed on all learners as they are recruited. Evaluation is limited to GNC set examinations and assessments of practice, as well as some, similar, school-generated assessments. The studies reported here argue strongly for the development of a model which caters much more for individual learner needs, problems and requirements at the planning, implementation and evaluation phases of the process.

Table 1: The Process model related to research, nursing and education

Process phase	Research	Nursing	Education
Assessment	Research question	Patient profile	Learner needs
Planning	Study design	Nursing care plan	Curriculum
Implementation	Data collection	Nursing practice	Educational and training programme
Evaluation	Analysis of data	Patient outcomes	Learner outcomes
Review	Research question	Patient profile	Learner needs

In the planning of a programme which includes the assessed needs and problems of the learners, as well as the requirements of the GNC and the clinical areas, the research findings of other studies are important. Those concerning relationships between school teaching and clinical experience show how the content and structure of the teaching as well as where it occurs can influence the progress of the learner (Bendall, 1975; Abdel-Al, 1975; Alexander, 1982; Gott, 1982). Those studies concerning the experiences of the learners on the ward, their perceptions of those who do or do not teach them, and the general climate in the learning situations indicate the importance of planning the who? when? where? and how? of the teaching in relation to the needs, problems and requirements of the learners (Lamonde, 1974; Fretwell, 1982). This also includes the preparation of those involved in education and training, with special reference to interpersonal as well as teaching skills. Increased sensitivity and interpersonal warmth on the part of those who have potential role involvement with the learner would seem to give them greater importance, and to give them greater influence over the kind of nursing that is learnt, and the kind of nurse that the learner eventually becomes.

Table 2: The phases of the Process Model as applied to the education system, with particular reference to nurse training

Phases of the Education Process

(1) Assess the learner's needs — identify problems
    as an individual
    as determined by the profession
    as determined by the service

(2) Plan the curriculum to meet these
    a timetable of experiences
    a programme of interventions
    criteria for evaluation

(3) Implement the programme
    recruit the learners
    institute the programme
    provide the interventions

(4) Evaluate the outcomes
    as identified in the assessment
    as laid down in the plan

(5) Review the programme in the light of the assessment
    for the individuals
    for groups

Another important aspect of the planning phase involves the setting up of objectives and criteria for evaluation, regarding the needs, problems and requirements of the learners. Extending these to include the monitoring of the learners' perceptions of the problems and progress as well as the more academic and practical assessments currently employed could usefully prevent problems developing into unmanageable situations. They could also help to explain failure to achieve practical and academic objectives. The educators could also benefit from the insights offered by the learners and from the input into the education process of an acknowledged active participation by them.

In conclusion it would seem that this last point is the most important one. For the studies presented here and those to which they refer indicate that nurse learners *will be* active in negotiating their progress through training, and in many instances will work things out for themselves. They will determine for themselves, on the basis of ideas and practices gained from their chosen, significant others (who well may be themselves or non-professionals) what kind of nurses they will become, and what kind of profession will exist in years to come. In many ways it can be argued that, at the present, learners become nurses in spite of the system, negotiating it afresh each time and making the same mistakes generation after generation. Without a research-based approach to nurse education, one that is related to learners' needs and constantly monitored and evaluated, there can be no real curricular development, nor can new schemes of training bring about real changes in the quality of nurses and the nursing that results.

References

Abdel-Al, H. 'Relating education to practice within a nursing context,' PhD Thesis, University of Edinburgh (1975)

Alexander, M.F. (1982) 'Integrating theory and practice in nursing, 1 and 2,' *Nursing Times, 78*, Occasional papers 17 and 18, 65-8, and 69-71

Bendall, E.R.D. (1975) *So You Passed, Nurse*, Royal College of Nursing, London

Fretwell, J.E. (1982) *Ward Learning and Teaching*, Royal College of Nursing, London

General Nursing Council for Scotland (1978) Schemes of training for the register of nurses, Edinburgh

Lamonde, N. (1974) *Becoming a Nurse*, Royal College of Nursing, London

Nurses, Midwives and Health Visitors Act (1979), HMSO, London

Report of the Committee on Nursing (Briggs Report, 1972), HMSO London

INDEX

For Product Safety Concerns and Information please contact our EU
representative GPSR@taylorandfrancis.com
Taylor & Francis Verlag GmbH, Kaufingerstraße 24, 80331 München, Germany

www.ingramcontent.com/pod-product-compliance
Lightning Source LLC
Chambersburg PA
CBHW070709190326
41458CB00004B/915